THE LUKIN LONGEVITY SYSTEM

The Guide To Staying Younger, Longer

NATASHA LUKIN

THE LUKIN LONGEVITY SYSTEM
The Guide to Staying Younger, Longer

ISBN 9781717885241

For general information on our other products
and services, please find our contact information online at
www.lukinlongevity.com

ABOUT THIS BOOK

"The Lukin Longevity System is a written phenomenon, not just a book. It is an easy to read piece of work with thoroughly well-selected material. The author uses smart metaphors and offers practical advice and exercises for readers to follow. It is a well-thought-out system and is worthwhile for anyone to consider for everyday use. It is especially interesting when you consider the author's personal achievements and her attitude to life."

— **Dr Boris Goloub, psychologist, MBBS, Grad Dip Prof Psych, Grad Dip App Sci (Psych)**

"A must-read longevity guide for anyone wanting to live a long and productive life. Read this book and learn from one of the best health and longevity experts who really walks her talk."

— **Dr Irina Webster, best-selling author of**
The Secret Energy of Your Body
www.dririnawebster.com

I started on my Lukin longevity program with Natasha Lukin on March 24, 2017. At that time I was going through tremendous stress with lots of unresolved issues in my life, and In our first 3-hour session we came up with a plan.

Since then, in 11 months I have lost 25kg and got my confidence back. My emotional state of mind improved and my physical body pays me off with lots of energy, vitality and it is shaping up beautifully.

The program requires discipline and the right tuning. Natasha is very easy going and your secrets are safe with her. She is so passionate about sharing her knowledge helping people in balancing their lives.

I love my results and my new mindset. I recommend Natasha to my friends regularly, because I sincerely believe her system works, and other people can have a similar experience to mine using Natasha's program and guidance.

— **Tasha Marchev, editor**
Bohemian Rhapsody Club and Magazine
www.bohemianrhapsodyclub.weebly.com

It seems that many of us like to share copybook maxims with our friends and relatives. After all, that is much easier to do than finding solutions for our own problems. Luckily, I have regular counselling sessions with Natasha Lukin, who has been able to not just offer me ready solutions but direct me towards having a fresh look at my problem and see it from a different angle. She knows how to listen and to hear and she sees the aspects of my problem that I have not been able to see, and when I see it too, I feel surprised how I could not notice it before when it was right in front of my nose!

Her system of mental exercises for opening your eyes to see your issues in a new light is unique in a way that it is simple and requires no special effort. You get results that are equally unique. Although her methods are very important, of no less importance is Natasha's personality as she is considerate and not pushy as an adviser. She knows how to create that necessary trusting connection with a client, allowing you to relax, and then your solutions come to you seemingly naturally.

I am glad that fate brought me in contact with Natasha Lukin and very grateful for all the time we spent together working on improving my various life situations. I wish Natasha all the best that she deserves for supporting people when they need help and understanding!

**— Alexander Rossini,
   business owner and travel consultant**

As a member of the Australasian Society of Lifestyle Medicine, I have a long-standing interest in healthy ageing. I am very much impressed by the Lukin Longevity System, offered by a scientist and health practitioner Natasha Lukin in her book. Her knowledge is insightful and put across in such a way that there can be no confusion. Not going deeper into science and research, It's simple, really. Who would want to live a miserable and uneventful 20 or 30 years when you can do things, see things and keep the spark burning? In my view, Natasha Lukin's book widens your horizons and provides you with practical steps on how to enjoy your Golden years to the full. This book should be handed out at the doctors' surgeries. I will definitely recommend it highly to my clients.

**— Marisha Rafaely, Naturopath, Master of Clinical Science,
   Healthy Ageing Medical Clinic, Melbourne**

A friend passed a copy of The Lukin Longevity System to me and explained that I owed it to myself to read it first and to judge it second. I'm so glad I did. I made some very simple changes to my life and I'm already feeling better. I am in my fifties and not in a 'bad place' to begin with but subconsciously I guess I had been thinking through getting old in a negative way. Natasha Lukin has made me reshuffle my thoughts towards approaching the 'autumnal years' and I'm now looking forward to it.

— Lena Frandi, accountant, New Zealand

As a naturopath myself I was particularly interested in Natasha Lukin's at-home remedies. In my practice I rely a lot on natural therapies. For many years I am collecting folk medicine recipes from around the world. I have already known some of Natasha's remedies, other are totally new ones. Thus, they become new additions to me collection. For example, her creak-free knee remedy 'Salvation for Your Knee Joints' would be helpful to many of my patients. However, first I give it a try myself, just to be sure how it works.

— Yael Kaminsky, Naturopath, Tel-Aviv, Israel

I could read it in a couple of nights and found it refreshingly different to all the other 'how to' books out there. You can tell it comes from a deep thinker and a doctor with an open mind and heart. It's easy to read and it should be a hand out at every doctors surgery.

— Anne Noonan, Forever Yoga, Certified Nutrition Coach, Diabetes Food Advisor

ACKNOWLEDGEMENT

Special thanks to:

Natalia Pakhomova, for the portrait of the Author on the front cover — **owlphotography.com.au**

Kate Romadinova — for design and management of my website and social media.

DEDICATION

I wish to dedicate this book with thanks to Drs Adriana and Tad James for their amazing courses in NLP and Time Line therapy that I have undertaken. The knowledge I learned there elevated my existing professional skills by helping me in clarifying, structuring and polishing my longevity system. The strategic psychological tools I accessed through them have become fundamental for my 'System of Beliefs' concept.

I am also very appreciative of Matt Lavars, an inspirational trainer in coaching at the Coaching Institute in Melbourne. Being such an enthusiastic and engaging presenter, he showed me how public speaking can be conducted at its best.

My sincere gratitude to Dr Andrew Cheng from Sydney Retina Clinic, a brilliant eye specialist who has been looking after my vision for many years, helping me to not succumb to losing my sight and remaining able to read and write, hopefully for many years ahead.

Finally, a special thank you to my publishing team at Best Seller Success, and especially to Joanne Harrison, my first encouraging reader. She was the one who brushed up my occasionally over-academic language and made it an easier and more engaging read.

And thank you to you as well, my brave, adventurous reader, for wanting a better, longer, healthier and more fulfilling life. I feel very honoured to be your guide on this journey.

FOREWORD

The oldest woman on record lived to be 122 – that's 60-plus years after people commonly retire. As our life expectancy increases, it seems only right we embrace our futures with as much enthusiasm and optimism as we did when they were blossoming. That is, to make goals, take care of ourselves and implement life systems that will ensure we reach a ripe age, enjoying good health and a fully functioning mind. Isn't it more pleasurable to imagine the next decades as fun and fulfilling rather than it being a decline into wrinkles and ill health?

Ask yourself, is there a greater gift to receive than the answers to longevity? Natasha Lukin's Longevity System is the culmination of a lifetime's findings. Natasha intermingles her personal experiences of a childhood growing up happily, healthily and harmoniously by the Black Sea in Georgia, with the academic knowledge from her studies in human biology and her investigations into the allied health fields.

As you well know, a gift isn't only appreciated by the receiver. Writing this book and sharing her passions and discoveries for making the most of life, whatever stage it is at, was highly pleasurable for Natasha. As a scientist, positive psychology practitioner, NLP life coach, health educator and writer there is only so much information you can keep to yourself, so sharing it all has truly enriched her life.

Negativity is a virus that plagues people of every culture. Its effects are devastating. However, there is a cure. This book is the anti-virus you need. Natasha Lukin treats the symptoms, providing a practical, step-by-step cure. Read it, apply it and your world will change.

— **Pat Mesiti,** International motivational speaker, the author of *Pathway to Prosperity: The 12 Steps to Financial Freedom, Staying Together Without Falling Apart: How to Thrive in a Modern-Day Relationship* and other best-selling books.

TABLE OF CONTENTS

About This Book. iii

Acknowledgement vii

Dedication ix

Foreword xi

About the Author. 1

Preface 5

SYSTEM OF BELIEFS

The Mystery of Ageing. 11

Age of the Brain. 14

Your Personal Beliefs About Ageing and
How to Think Youthful Thoughts 16

STEP 1 — Identify Your Beliefs About Age,
Ageing and Longevity 17

STEP 2 — Ask Yourself: How Do These Beliefs Affect
My Life or How Would They Affect My Future?. 19

STEP 3 — Trace the Origin of Your Limiting Beliefs. 20

STEP 4 — Replace Your Limiting Beliefs with
New, Empowering Ones 20

STEP 5 — What is Holding Us Back from Fulfilling
Our Promise to Ourselves? 25

STEP 6 — How Catherine the Great Programmed
Her Mind in Seven Steps 27

Brain Hygiene 29

Keep Your Memory Green 31

Trust Your Memory 34

SYSTEM OF GOALS

How to be S.M.A.R.T. 41

Focus: How Your Dream Becomes a Goal 43

The Pen is Mightier Than the Sword 46

Why Some Vision Boards Work and Others Don't. 47

Excuses and Other Calamities 50

Dealing with Problems 54

The Logic Mind Assumes, While the
Subconscious Mind Knows. 54

The Secret of Rocambole. 55

How to Go from Knowing What to Do ...
to Actually Doing It 57

Other Tips for Doing Things 62

SYSTEM OF ACTIONS

The Secret of Looking Young. 65

Clear Vision 66

Say Goodbye to Lines and Sagging Skin 68

Facial Expressions 70

The Mona Lisa Smile 73

Fitness for Health and Enjoyment .74

How to Make Sensible Choices About Nutrition 81

Water—The Greatest Healer of All 90

Nine Signs You're Not Drinking Enough Water 92

A Myth About Salt 94

Sleepless at Night 95

Memory and Mnemonic Training. 100

Natural Remedies. 104

Bicarbonate of Soda—A Miracle Mineral 106

More about salt 107

Iodine 108

Salvation for Your Knee Joints 109

Seven recipes for Brain Vessel Cleansing. 110

The Easiest Remedy to Rejuvenate
Your Body in 40 Days 113

Great News on Coughing and Chocolate 115

Garlic Husk—Look Younger for Longer 115

A Killer of Extra Kilos 117

The Plant of "Eternal Youth" 118

Parsley Lotion 119

Flax Seeds Against Parasites 120

The Healing Power of Coriander 120

Golden Age—The Secret of Longevity 123

ABOUT THE AUTHOR

I am Natasha Lukin, a scientist, positive psychology practitioner, NLP life coach, health educator and writer.

When one has been living long enough, working productively and gaining an ample scope of life experiences, as I have, there comes a time when you may feel a strong need to share your knowledge 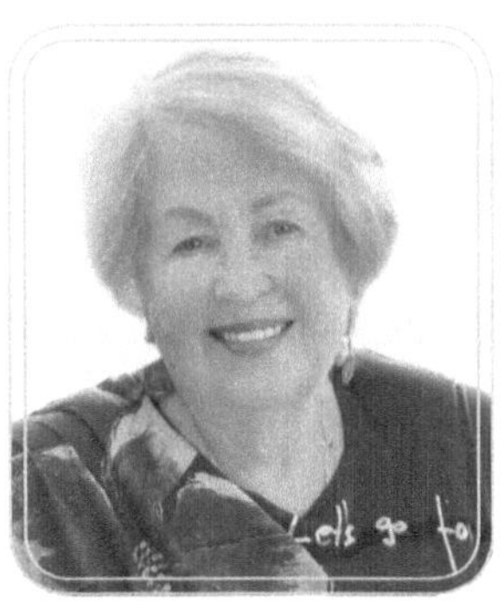 and skills—that is exactly what I am doing with this book. The process of giving is very rewarding, and I hope that this book will support you, my readers, in your search for the answers to some of life's biggest questions.

I created this Longevity System program based on my extensive experience in allied health fields, my knowledge of human biology and the environment I grew up in. My mother was a prominent scientist with a doctorate related to human development and my grandmother was a dentist, while my great uncle was a professor of botany and the author of numerous books on medicinal herbs and plants. Even my mother-in-law and step-mother were both paediatricians so, from a very young age, I was around a lot of talk about health, medicine and human development.

I was born and bred in the former USSR, more precisely the city of Moscow, but I grew up in Georgia, in a pretty town called

Sukhumi, right by the Black Sea. It was a magical childhood, filled with blossoming magnolia, camellia, oleanders, wattle trees, pyramidal cypresses, fresh fruit and veg. They were all natural—or as we say now, organic!

The Black Sea supplied us with the yummiest fish such as mullet, horse mackerel and flounder. They would be unloaded from the fishermen's boats straight into our kitchen. We used kerosene devices for cooking and boiling water. We didn't know any better and we were happy with what we had. We would ride our bikes and go for a swim in the sea with no supervision. We collected mussels on the beach and ate them. We had an excellent school and wonderful teachers whose names I will remember forever. The society was multicultural—nobody cared whether you were ethnic Russian, Georgian, Ukrainian, Jewish, Greek, Abkhazian, Chechen or anything else.

> **"I created this Longevity System program based on my extensive experience in allied health fields, my knowledge of human biology and the environment I grew up in."**

Well, it's all long gone now and my heart aches to look upon the ruins of Sukhumi. Because of bad blood between nationals, hundreds perished in the war and thousands fled their homes, leaving all their belongings behind. It was so incredibly sad.

After graduating from school, I made my way to Moscow. Because of my excellent school records (I was awarded a gold medal—20 grams of pure 14-carat gold!) I was accepted into the prestigious Moscow State Lomonosoff University. My fields of study included various aspects of biology such as human physiology, biochemistry, biophysics, genetics, epidemiology, psychology and many others. My studies, both in schools and tertiary institutions were very in-depth. Requirements were extremely high and there was absolutely no concept of having fun while you studied. Following five-and-a-half years of hard work, assessments and exams, I was awarded my degree. I had to present my graduation essay to the commission, defending my points against specially-appointed opponents.

My first job was a junior scientist in a biochemistry laboratory at the major trauma and orthopaedic hospital. However, I discovered my natural calling was more oriented to presentation and writing—working with people, not just Petri dishes and electrophoreses. After becoming a scientist in human biology, I realised that I didn't want as much to do with science as I wanted to write about it and implement my knowledge by educating and enlightening readers and listeners.

After a while, I became a journalist specialising in science, health and psychology. I was published in many newspapers and magazines and then worked as a reporter and scriptwriter for television in Moscow. My first few published books, written in Russian, were on popular health and the history of medicine themes that helped me to establish myself as an author. In 1992, I was offered a part-time job as a Russian language tutor at the University of Melbourne, which led me to relocate to Australia. Soon after arrival, I enrolled at RMIT to study interpreting and translating.

After getting my certificates, I became a NAATI-accredited interpreter and translator, working for a number of organisations such as the Cancer Council of Victoria, Mercy Hospital, community health centres and also for private businesses and individuals. In 1998, I wrote *The Bride from Moscow*, a romantic thriller novel, written in English, published in the UK, with a second edition published in 2010. Unfortunately, due to not having a marketing machine behind the book, it didn't do that well.

After giving up on writing for a while, I decided to turn my attention to an opportunity that appeared to me totally by chance in 2008. At the age of 67, I entered into the unknown territory of owning a small business, by opening a Shapemaster Feel Good Studio in Canberra. Here I had a chance to realise my potential as a human biologist and psychologist. For seven years, I helped my clients—the majority being women aged 45 or above—to get into better shape, not just physically but also emotionally. In 2016, I concluded the seven-year term by selling my studio to a doctor and turned my attention to positive psychology.

In the last couple of years, I've done a community mediation course in Canberra, and a number of online psychology courses and intensive neuro-linguistic programming studies with doctors Tad and Adriana James in Sydney. I received *my four qualifying certificates as* an NLP life coach, NLP practitioner, Time Line therapist and hypnotist. Now, this is my passion and my business as well. NLP is an amazing discipline that uncovers new pathways to help people learn problem-solving skills in any area of their life, whether it's relationships, family, children, career, finance, health, personal development or spirituality.

By writing this book, I wish to send a message to my readers—life is an adventure, a chore and a gift to enjoy. And our age has nothing to do with that. What we do with our life is up to us at any stage of this journey, whether we're young, old or somewhere in between.

PREFACE

"When the mind is thinking, it is talking to itself."

—Plato

Firstly, thank you for purchasing this book. I hope you find the encouragement to live your life to the full for many years to come.

Stop counting your passport years. Stop living and acting according to the date that is printed in there—just stop it! We have all the time in the world to fill it with all those fabulous things, events, discoveries and fantasies that can be made a reality. But you know what many of us do instead, don't you? We voluntarily invite all these so-called "age-related" conditions into our life. We send signals to both our conscious and unconscious minds that we are ready to get old.

We all know it doesn't have to be that way. We've all heard of people climbing the Sydney Harbour Bridge in their eighties, getting married in their seventies and starting new ventures after turning sixty? In fact, I am one of those people! I started my first small business with zero experience at the age of 67. I had moderate success and sold it aged 75.

Of course, all of this is relative and comparable. I am not suggesting you be silly or unrealistic, nor am I saying do everything you did (or didn't do but wanted to do) in your youth. Your body dictates that you observe your limits and act wisely with some adjustment and modification. However, that should not stop you—no way!

Rejoice constantly that you are still able to set foot on grass, admire blue skies and fluffy clouds, and let the rain stream its holy waters over you—provided you have a decent raincoat! While the body's agility slows down, with a clever mind you can still achieve tremendous results using other avenues and making smarter decisions.

Right now, you might be thinking to yourself, "Natasha, I know all of that—nothing you have written so far surprises me." I'm not delusional. Of course, I realise that whatever I or other experts say, you've probably heard it or read it somewhere before. I have dedicated a whole chapter to the 100-mile gap between "I know" and "I do". As Cormac McCarthy wrote in his book *All the Pretty Horses*, "Between the wish and the thing, the world lies waiting."

> **"I believe this is a great time in our lives, where we get to take a good, long look at what we want, what's been missing in our lives and what we still hope to achieve."**

Did you know that each period of our life has its markers? Markers for the young include growing up, learning and trying different things, experiencing first love, making friends, being bold, brave and silly and believing we are invincible. Meanwhile, a marker for adult life, in a stereotypical sense, would be finding a job, being promoted, getting married, having children, being responsible for your family, colleagues, community and even the world! This phase can last for 30-40 years. Then a very new and different one begins.

Retirement may be looming—although the goal posts seem to be continually moving on that one—the kids are all grown up and have flown the coop. You may be married, divorced or even widowed. Then what? Now that we are all living longer, we need to create a new marker. What could the next 20, 30 or even 40 years bring?

I believe this is a great time in our lives, where we get to take a good, long look at what we want, what's been missing in our lives and what we still hope to achieve. That means setting goals, taking good care of your health and getting more out of life every day. Whether you are one of the lucky ones and can retire, or you need to continue working, this is a special time in your life and only you get to say how it turns out.

You will find a lot of useful advice, stunning discoveries and helpful recommendations within these pages, ready to support you to create your best marker yet—enjoy!

"Be Transformed By The Renewing of Your Mind"

The Bible – Romans 12:2

SYSTEM OF BELIEFS

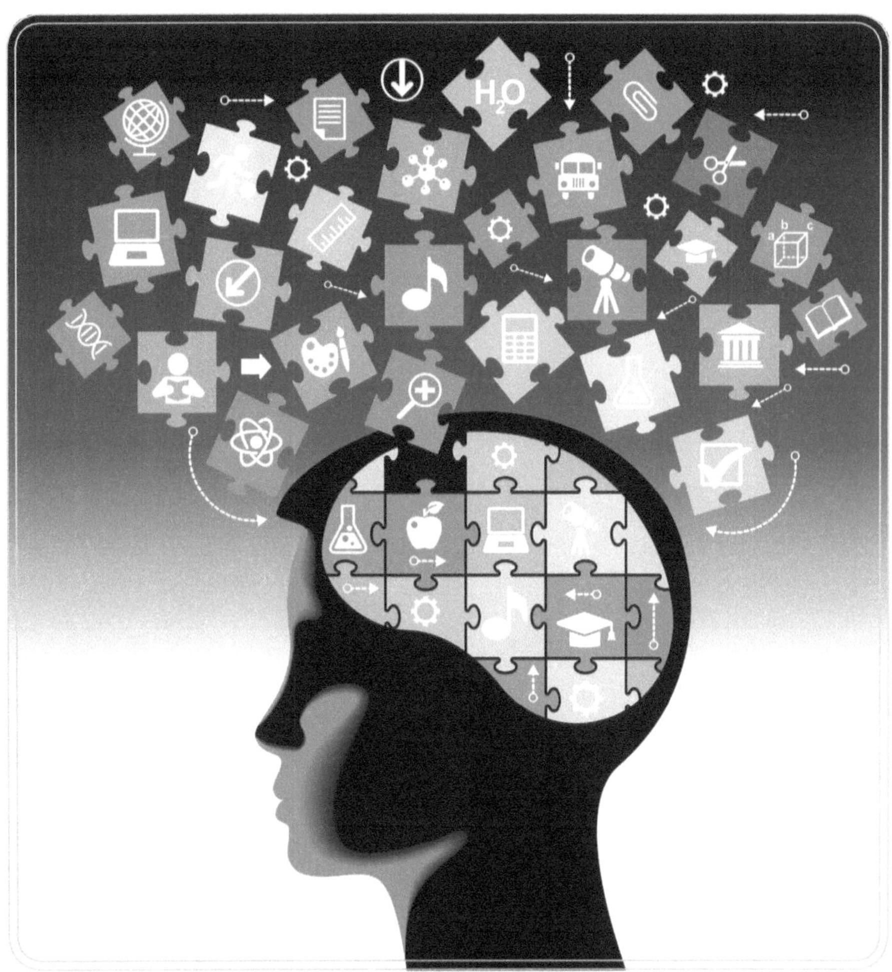

The Mystery of Ageing

*"To live is the rarest thing in the world.
Most people exist, that is all."*

—Oscar Wilde

Let's look at the keywords: *age, ageing* and *longevity*. Longevity as a concept is quite fluid these days. The longest living person on Earth was Madam Jeanne Louise Calment, a French super-centenarian who verifiably lived to the age of 122 years and 164 days.

However, Dr Aubrey David Nicholas Jasper de Grey, a biomedical gerontologist and the author of a sensational book called *Ending Ageing*, made an astonishing statement that humans can live for a thousand years.

De Grey claimed the "indefinite postponement of ageing may be within sight" back in 2002. In the 15 years since, his reputation among gerontologists—scientists concerned with ageing—has gone from being one of ridicule to one of the most powerful and respected in the industry. In 2009, the 53-year-old scientist founded the public non-profit SENS—Strategies for Engineered Negligible Senescence. Through his foundation, De Grey has drawn a roadmap to defeat biological ageing.

> **"To know your age, you look at the date in your passport. To evaluate ageing, you look at the condition of the person."**

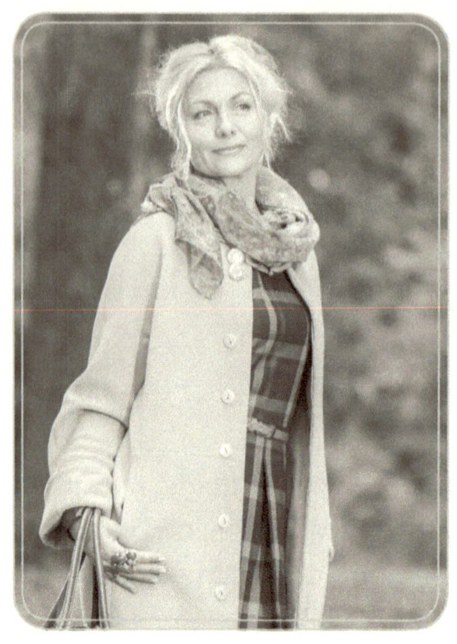

What he meant is that, with time, any process in a living organism could make and accumulate errors—for example, in cell division or mutations. External damage could also interfere with smooth body processes. His point is that advances in the bio-technologies of damage repair, including the replacement of body parts, stem cell therapies and similar discoveries would significantly increase the longevity threshold.

Of course, De Grey and other researchers are not aiming to increase our lifespan to a thousand years, as that could create an incredible population crisis. They don't believe we're going to live forever—nor should we. The great majority of longevity scientists are not looking for immortality but for healthy ageing. They want to give us a healthier, longer life followed by compressed morbidity—a quick and painless death. This is all very encouraging.

Let's get back to ageing. How do we perceive these notions? For some people, they sound like they are about old age. About growing old, battling illnesses, gradually becoming frail and senile. The problem is, when we think this way, we are submissively inviting these experiences into our lives like lambs to the slaughter.

Fortunately, not everyone agrees. Other people see it differently and make the distinction in simple terms—age is a number, *ageing* is a condition. To know your age, you look at the date in your passport. To evaluate ageing, you look at the condition of the person. Age is about progressing in years, while ageing relates to the performance of our body and mind. We cannot change our age, but we can change our physical, mental and psychological condition. Lifestyle optimisation is very much in fashion right now, and rightly so.

To elaborate more and emphasise that growing old is not a linear process, imagine a young man in his twenties, recovering from broken bones, taking his first unbalanced steps, supported by a nurse, when each step gives him arthritis-like pain in his joints—do you think he feels like a cheerful youngster or more like a sixty-year-old invalid?

The point is we associate certain conditions with age. However, in real terms, it's nothing like that. Recovering after having their appendix removed, a 25-year-old would feel more like they were 45 due to the anaesthetic and general after-effects of surgery. Some women experience early menopause. They might be in their thirties, but their physical experience would be more like that of a fifty-year-old woman. So, if we assign conditions to a certain age you will see it is not a linear progression, but more up and down, backwards and forwards or even a zig-zag pattern. Therefore, growing old and ageing are not the same.

We cannot do anything about the progression of years, but we can do a lot about the quality of our life as we get older. The umbrella word is anti-ageing—that includes a variety of aspects, ideas, attitudes and an ample scope of actions and measures to get more out of life. The foremost principle for those who are not willing to succumb to ageing is to start living anew. We live in a fantastic era, where those old, stagnant ideas go out of the window and are replaced with a slogan—life is for living, no matter your age.

Age of the Brain

So, we already talked about your biological age, but how about the age of your brain? It is well-known that your biological age does not convey any real information about either your health condition nor your physical potentials—for example, the speed of your reactions.

It is also not particularly helpful to estimate someone's age by their looks. Sometimes, I look at a person and think they are in their forties but then I learn that they're in their early thirties. This also works the other way around. Someone might say, "This woman isn't a day over 35," but it turns out she just celebrated her big five-0 last week. Thus, it doesn't make sense to be guided by your date of birth. It does not reflect your real age. So, how do we know your true age? No doubt, you have some idea—let's check to see whether we think the same. To establish the *true* age of a person one normally checks three parameters:

- The endurance of the heart under physical stress.

- Flexibility of joints.

- Speed of reaction.

All the above parameters are used to define the biological age of a person. However, they don't include the characteristics of irreversibility, which means that every parameter could either change for the worse with age or, equally, could change for the better.

We need to stop being guided by limiting beliefs about the so-called inevitability of ageing and irreversibility of age-related changes.

The main parameter among those three is the speed of our reactions, which relates to our brain. By training our brain to increase the speed of our reactions, our heart and joint parameters automatically improve. This means that, by training our brain, not just those but many other important biological parameters can improve. As a result, our biological system rejuvenates.

The twenty-first century has been announced as the century of biology. We are lucky that, right now, many discoveries are being made or are in the pipeline to help us live longer and more productively. However, it doesn't mean we just sit with our arms crossed and wait for them to be delivered.

Scientists and researchers do their job but we must also do ours. Then our cumulative results will bring us experiences like never before: feeling younger, happier and healthier against our previous limiting beliefs and expectations. It's a fantastic time for seniors and for younger people thinking about their future. We used to be bombarded with limiting beliefs about ageing, but we need to get rid of them, like old barnacles that have been scraped off the underside of a ship, to allow it to begin sailing again.

> **"Our future starts today. It is our choice how we want it to be—no one else's."**

Our future starts today. It is our choice how we want it to be—no one else's. If you need encouragement, advice, support and a friendly hand, rest assured, you've found it.

Your Personal Beliefs About Ageing and How to Think Youthful Thoughts

The media today seems to be rushing to offer everyone the latest advice on how to look younger and live longer. Have you ever wondered what really helps us to live a long, healthy and youthful life? Well, you are not alone—that is why I have made it my mission to find the answers to these questions and many more about ageing and longevity, and why I created *The Lukin Longevity System.*

Did you even know that you had beliefs about age, ageing and longevity? Sometimes, we are so caught up in our lives that we simply don't realise that we carry these beliefs around with us, never consciously questioning them. They become more than just beliefs—they become our *truth,* unquestioned or even unnoticed. Unfortunately, they also play havoc with our experience of life. Have you ever stopped and asked yourself, "What do I believe about ageing and longevity?" Doing so is the first step to staying younger and living longer.

Your mind is like a computer platform. Our beliefs and preconceptions are like computer programs running in our brain. Therefore, they can be modified—or deleted. Those programs have been installed there, often unconsciously, as "gifts" from parents, teachers or society. You may even have some installed that behave more like viruses. On that subject, there is a remarkable book called *Viruses of the Mind* by Richard Dawkins.

So, how can we uninstall the programs that represent our limiting beliefs and wipe out these viruses? Firstly, let's get back to definitions of age, ageing and longevity:

Age is easy to define—you take out your passport or birth certificate and you can see your date of birth. Then deduct the current year and bingo: that is your "age". As each year passes, you become one year older.

Ageing is a condition of your body, your mind and how you live your life. It is proven that humans can live up to 120-140 years before there is any kind of rapid decline physically and mentally. Unfortunately, when most people turn 50-60 years old they start telling themselves they are getting old, saying things like, "At my age, I'll start getting arthritis soon."

Longevity means "long life" but it doesn't have to mean just living for a long time, especially as most see that as suffering without any enjoyment due to their body failing them. Longevity can mean living a long time with vitality and all of your faculties fully intact. Whether we're turning twenty or eighty, our fears about getting older can have a stressful and limiting impact on how we feel about ourselves, our relationships and what we see as possible in our lives.

STEP 1
Identify Your Beliefs About Age, Ageing and Longevity

What are some common limiting beliefs about age, ageing and longevity?

- I can only date people my own age.

- People at a certain age don't do this sort of thing.

- Women over forty shouldn't grow their hair long.

- You can't teach an old dog new tricks.

- Ageing leads to loneliness.

- Ageing eliminates your libido.
- There is no point in trying to get fit—it's all downhill after forty.
- Dementia is to be expected with old age.
- Older workers are less productive than younger workers.
- The body degrades/breaks down with age.
- Old people are boring and forgetful.
- Old people are grouchy and cantankerous.
- My mother and my grandmother had [insert disease/illness] so I will get it.

To discover some of your limiting beliefs about ageing, complete or answer the below statements and questions:

- I am too old to:
- It's too late for me to learn:
- Where do I limit myself in my life due to my beliefs about age?
- What do I believe about ageing?
- Which of the above "common limiting beliefs about ageing" do I identify with?
- If you have an ailment, what do you tell yourself about it?
- I'm worried about getting old because:
- What does society tell you about ageing?
- What am I saying or doing to myself that is holding me back, related to ageing?

STEP 2
Ask Yourself: How Do These Beliefs Affect My Life or How Would They Affect My Future?

Do you hold yourself back, believing that what you can do is limited by your age? You shouldn't go after that promotion, learn that new hobby or start that new venture because people your age "shouldn't do that"?

Have you heard of the term "self-fulfilling prophecy"? A sociologist named Robert K. Merton created this term in 1948 to describe "a false definition of the situation evoking a new behaviour, which makes the originally false conception come true". In other words, the prediction we make at the start of something affects our behaviour in such a way that we make that possibility a reality.

> **"When you know what your limiting beliefs are, how they affect you and where they came from, you'll be able to go about removing them, so you can stay younger, longer!"**

This is how powerful our beliefs are. If you believe you are forgetful, you will be. Occasionally, we all forget things like our keys or glasses. However, if you berate yourself for it, you reinforce that belief about yourself. Those things will start happening more often and become a habit because you see yourself as a forgetful person in your own mind.

So, how do you break this vicious cycle?

STEP 3
Trace the Origin of Your Limiting Beliefs

Now, you won't always be able to do this but a lot of the time it really helps to get clarity about where your beliefs came from. You weren't born with them. These are programs you have installed along the way. We normally begin to create our belief system around our teenage years, but they can creep in even earlier. Who told you about this new "computer program" you should install? Did you read it in an article?

Maybe you had a conversation with your neighbours and they were very convincing—they had a lot of evidence to prove their *belief* was the *truth*. Was it something your parents repeated regularly? Did you watch a news segment on TV?

When you know what your limiting beliefs are, how they affect you and where they came from, you'll be able to go about removing them, so you can stay younger, longer!

STEP 4
Replace Your Limiting Beliefs with
New, Empowering Ones

You can find various techniques on how to do this online and in books. The method I'm going to offer you here I use myself and with my clients. It is simple, and it *works*.

Start with writing down three of your old, limiting beliefs. For example:

- ➡ "I believe ageing equals illness."

- ➡ "I will look ridiculous if I go dancing."

> "I am not supposed to take any risks—that could be dangerous at my age."

Write new beliefs in the present tense or use progressive tense, whichever feels better.

> "I enjoy feeling healthy and vital as I age."

> "I don't care what they think about me going dancing."

> "I believe that ageing is an opportunity for new experiences."

Now you have listed your old beliefs and created new ones to replace them, you need to do the mental work and use your imagination to make the change. Bring your first old belief up on your mental screen and see it clearly in your mind's eye, like it's written on a whiteboard. Pick up a 'wet sponge' and start erasing it from right to left, letter by letter. Once you have erased the entire belief, make sure the image is completely blank. If there are any letters or even shadows left, repeat erasing until there is nothing left.

Take a whiteboard marker to your board, preferably bright red, and start writing from left to right. Read your letters aloud as you create your new belief. Observe and admire your writing and feel the energy of it circulating through your body. Illuminate the background.

If you have difficulty picturing your belief in your mind's eye, you may also make your affirmations in writing. It is still an effective method but takes a bit longer. Write out your new belief on a paper a hundred times a day. Keep doing that for at least twenty days in a row without missing even one day. The reason why people feel their affirmations don't work is that they're not repeating them properly. Communicating your desires to a higher power requires persistence, a fact well-established by people who practice spirituality.

Make sure when you write it out that you imagine how it feels to believe this new thought. How does your life look? What are you doing? What actions are you taking? What is showing up in your life now that you hold this new belief?

Other great ways to use your affirmations are:

- Repeat your affirmations during the day, when you are driving, exercising or standing in a queue. You can repeat them out loud where appropriate, or silently.

- Write them on a piece of card. Put them on your bathroom mirror or around the house in any place where you will see them.

- Recording your affirmations on a device, such as a smartphone, is a great way to embed them in your mind. You can listen to them throughout your day and even when you are falling asleep—that can work wonders!

Here is a great story about an older gentleman who was lucky enough to cross paths with a youthful-minded person that got his life back on track by encouraging him to think new thoughts. Meet Peter and Lilian.

> **"Here is a great story about an older gentleman who was lucky enough to cross paths with a youthful-minded person."**

Peter took a last glance in the mirror to check his looks. Not bad-looking. A real gentleman, with decent posture for a 65-year-old. Peter was ready for his date. He had spent hours online in search of a woman to grow old with. It had become second nature for him to check the dating sites as soon as he woke up in the morning—were there any new ladies? This had been his morning routine since he had realised that old age was catching up with him.

He didn't feel too bad or have any health problems but by his age, he felt he was supposed to have some. He would think to himself, "I must be prepared." He needed a spouse, a partner, a companion—now, while he was still okay. Someone to grow old with, so it wasn't all so scary. He'd always felt that inevitability of decline because old age meant being sick and sore joints. "That is how nature works," Peter would tell himself.

He liked her picture. There was something lovely about her curly hair, all in disarray, and her eyes—were they really that blue? They exchanged a couple of messages. Before Peter knew it, they had arranged a date and today was the day! When he arrived at the café she was already there and waved to him from the table. Her smile was inviting—he felt good about this date. He started with the usual conversation and since he had been lied to so many times by women about their age, he decided to ask her directly.

"So, how old are you, Lilian?"

"I am ageless," she smiled softly. "Why would either of us need to know? Does it have any meaning?"

He took it as a joke.

"Angels are ageless," he said, "but we mere mortals must count our years."

"Must we?" she repeated. "What for?"

"Because…" he stumbled—suddenly, he didn't know how to reply. "Because we need to be prepared accordingly, don't you think?"

"What kind of preparation are you talking about?" she replied.

"Well … to prepare for the age-related illnesses that will inevitably come knocking, becoming frail and senile!" he exclaimed, feeling very certain about his comments. "My lady, you can't just bury your head in the sand. It's a fact of life!"

"Oh, well," she said, "I've got my own preparation. When I get up in the morning I greet the sun and the sky with a smile. I thank my body for being alive and healthy and I look forward to another wonderful day. I might meet with friends and go to the movies or visit my grandchildren. I love to go for walks along the Esplanade or do a bit of shopping. I drink hot chocolate and eat sweets. I go and see my hairdresser for a modern, new haircut. When I can afford it, on the spur of the moment, I might fly somewhere for a few days, whatever takes my fancy. And I don't feel guilty about my pleasures. I live my life to the fullest!"

Peter was disappointed that she had turned out to be a frivolous, silly woman. "What about men?" he said sternly. "Do you go with them on the spur of the moment too?"

"Not really," she whispered. "For that, I need to fall in love. To be in love is so wonderful, don't you agree?"

His irritation grew. How could she be so irresponsible, so flippant about the problems that accompany old age?

"What is your preparation then?" she asked, with a sincere curiosity. "How do you do it?"

He really wanted to put her in her place. But suddenly, he didn't know what to say. How was he preparing? By spending all his time being preoccupied with future problems that might not even occur? Thinking about getting sick and how he would cope with it? And then, how he would die? All this gloom and doom was in such stark contrast to her light, airy attitude to life that he suddenly envied her. Maybe if he changed his way of thinking his life would be more interesting, more fulfilling even more thrilling?

Observing his facial expressions, she said sympathetically, "You are still wearing a uniform. I mean, the uniform of prescribed ideas. Someone else's beliefs, lots of dos and don'ts. Take it off. It's stopping you from living!"

"Lillian," Peter blurted out, "could I join you on your walk along the Esplanade and then finish with a hot chocolate in Acland Street, please?'"

Her jingle-bell laughter was warm and light. "Sunday morning at 10 am in St. Kilda would be fabulous—but we will start with the hot chocolate!"

"Thank goodness," he thought to himself. "I really need to lighten up. I don't want someone to get old with, I want to live life with someone. This woman might be the one I was looking for all along."

STEP 5
What is Holding Us Back from Fulfilling Our Promise to Ourselves?

I wish to touch on another aspect of reprogramming the mind. How many people promise themselves the following?

- "Tomorrow, I will quit smoking."

- "From Monday, I'll stop eating after six."

- "Next month, I'll enrol in the gym."

➔ "Next week, I'll stop aimlessly trawling the internet."

The majority of these promises get broken more-or-less immediately, if not sooner. We commonly think it's about a lack of willpower, but it's not. Dr Maxwell Maltz, the author of *Psycho-Cybernetics: A New Way to Get More Living Out of Life* was the first medical scientist who discovered the real reason we fail to fulfil our best intentions. Our self-image is what defines our boundaries of possibilities.

Dr Maltz discovered that if our goals contradict our limiting beliefs about who we are, what we are able to do and what we are not, we have no chance of realising our intentions. Limiting beliefs constitute our opinion of ourselves. Unfortunately, these thoughts do not appear on the surface. Our conscious mind doesn't even know how we really think of ourselves.

> **"Our self-image is what defines our boundaries of possibilities."**

Dr Maltz stated that if our self-image features our stagnant feelings that we are not capable of certain actions, no contradicting intentions can ever be fulfilled. Therefore, following this theory, we need to evaluate whether there is something in our mind that is preventing us from achieving a particular goal. In this book, we are talking about the anti-ageing that can be jeopardised by our own limiting beliefs. The most common labels are:

➔ "I'm not good enough."

➔ "I'm useless."

➔ "I never achieve anything."

They are so deeply embedded in your subconscious mind that you are practically unaware of them. Unless we consciously search for these negative ideas about ourselves and work to change them around, no power in the world can help us to follow our plans through.

Dr Maltz's *Psycho-Cybernetics* postulates that if we don't address these issues, and our self-image is low, we will get stuck in a continuing pattern of limiting beliefs. Your opinion of yourself pre-determines what you can and cannot allow yourself to do. That opinion is, of course, an unconscious one, and that is why you never win the battle. No amount of willpower will prevail unless you change your beliefs.

The solution is pretty simple: if what you promise to yourself is in conflict with your unconscious opinion of yourself then you are doomed to fail. Check your limiting beliefs and reprogram your mind before deciding on your intentions.

STEP 6
How Catherine the Great Programmed Her Mind in Seven Steps

Catherine the Great, born as Princess Sophie of Anhalt-Zerbst to German nobility, was Empress of Russia from 1762 until 1796, the country's longest-ruling female monarch. Under her reign, Russia grew larger and stronger in cultural and military terms and became recognised as one of the great powers in Europe.

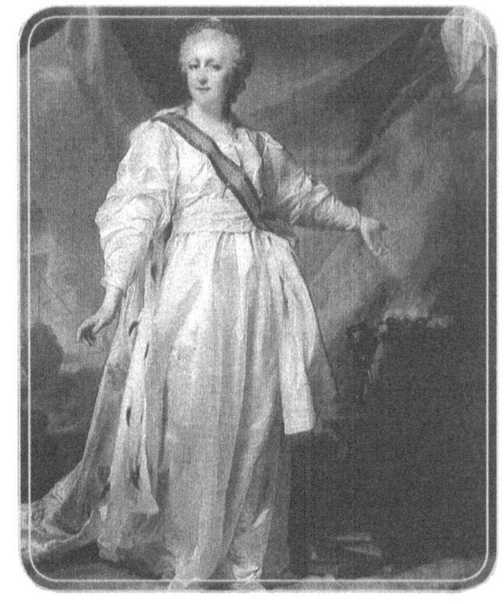

The story goes that Catherine the Great developed her special approach to decision-making on the advice of her mentor, Archbishop Simon Teodorsky. He taught her to not let any doubts interfere and to trust that her decisions were always the best. Their method from nearly three centuries ago is perfectly in-sync with our modern positive psychology techniques. So, here it is—the great monarch's secret, step by step.

1. Drink a glass of water in slow gulps.

2. Stand up, keeping your back straight. Inhale very slowly and as deeply as possible.

3. Make three rounding shoulder movements to immediately decrease your stress. Take time to feel the difference and hold on to it.

4. Repeat to yourself ten times, "My decisions are always the correct ones."

5. Be fully engrossed in it, following every word in your mind. Feel the power of those words, not just mentally but in your body as well.

6. As soon as you have said it the tenth time, make your decision. Don't look for logic, trust yourself—feel no fear.

7. The very first thought that crosses your mind in relation to the decision you are trying to make will always be the correct one.

What was good enough for the empress is good enough for us! In case it all seems too simple and you have doubts that it really works, here it is explained using a more current psychological perspective. When you drink a glass of water, due to its electrolyte properties, it saturates your body with quality energy and makes you stronger. When you take a deep breath, as you exhale, you enter a regime of steady, physiologically-correct, rhythmic breathing. This makes you even stronger and your heart chakra opens. This is a very powerful generator of both biological and psychic energy.

When you meaningfully and consciously repeat a phrase like, "My decisions are always correct," you create a protective mental screen against a doubtful phrase like, "What if I'm wrong?" that could direct your thoughts to your left hemisphere where the logic resides. Instead, your brainwave activity should go to the right hemisphere, reaching your unconscious mind. That is how the positive affirmation becomes a program. The program then commands your unconscious mind to find a way to implement your decision.

Brain Hygiene

As we discussed, our beliefs reside in our two minds, conscious and unconscious. Our brain—just like any other organ—needs maintenance and to be kept active, so it doesn't get rusty. For optimal functionality, our brain needs support from other parts of the body.

Let's talk a little about our brain hygiene. Blood circulation is paramount for the brain to be healthy. Tremendous amounts of blood circulate daily through our brain's blood vessels. If the blood doesn't flow freely, our brain activity is hindered. The quality of your blood depends on its saturation with

> **"When you drink a glass of water, due to its electrolyte properties, it saturates your body with quality energy and makes you stronger."**

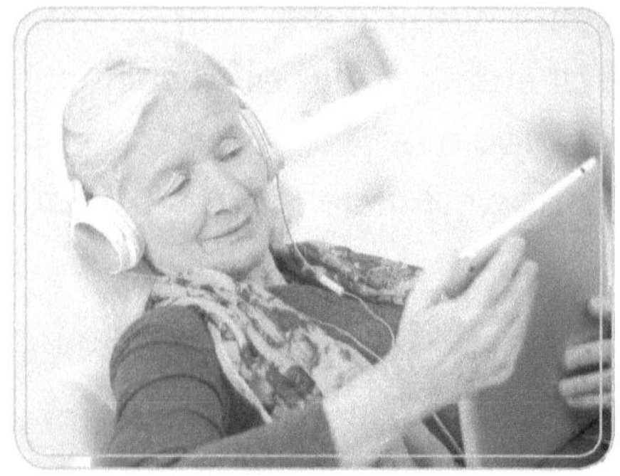

oxygen, as well as its components for which your doctor, from time to time, will send you for a blood test. If this test shows any sort of abnormality, it is up to your doctor to find a treatment. However, you are also in charge.

Always remember to get fresh air, take short breaks, open windows, go for a stroll, clean the atmosphere in your home and workplace. Eliminate clutter and make sure you keep up with the housework. Make sure you get a good night's sleep. Sleep deprivation is damaging to our brain activity and memory. We all know how much brighter we feel after an uninterrupted quality sleep. Give your brain a dose of oxygen and a good night's rest. Do you like Sudoku, puzzles or crosswords? This is gymnastics for your brain and memory, as well as being a pleasant and entertaining pastime. Pay attention to how your brain feels.

"Show your brain that you care and be rewarded with clearer thoughts and faster reactions as well as better moods."

British scientists from the University of Exeter and Royal College of Physicians in London analysed data from 17,000 seniors who were subjected to cognitive tests over a number of years. The results revealed that people who loved crosswords reliably demonstrated a higher level of concentration, attention to detail and better memory. We pay far more attention to our brawn than our brain. Show your brain that you care and be rewarded with clearer thoughts and faster reactions as well as better moods.

Keep Your Memory Green

Memory
All alone in the moonlight
I can smile at the old days
I was beautiful then
I remember
The time I knew what happiness was
Let the memory live again.

— From *Cats*

"Remember that beautiful girl, she's a movie star. You know … she's got that airy-fairy look—blonde, slender, tall. What's her name? She was in *Sliding Doors*."

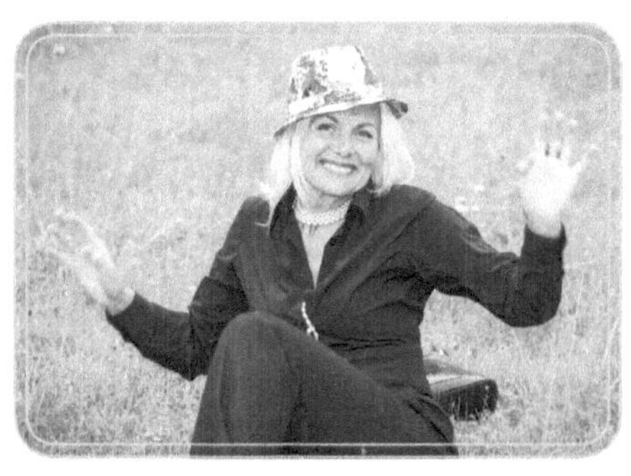

"Oh sure, of course, I know who you're talking about. Just give me a second. I see her clearly now, right in front of my eyes, but her name…"

"How annoying! Now I will be tortured for hours."

"Me too!"

"Wait … it's Gwyneth Paltrow!"

"Of course, Gwyneth Paltrow. How funny, I can almost feel the gears shifting in my head trying to figure that one out."

"Yep, same for me, it feels like I'm sifting through a filing cabinet and it takes time to find the right record back there."

I bet you're saying, "Been there, done that!" Me too. We all remember a lot, but we also forget a lot. As Cormac McCarthy noted in his prize-winning novel *The Road*, "You forget what you want to remember, and you remember what you want to forget."

Here's a question for you: Whose life is easier—someone with a poor memory or someone with a phenomenal memory?

Poor memory is a drag. It limits your actions, makes you uncertain about yourself. It can be embarrassing or even dangerous, like when you can't remember if you turned off the gas or unplugged the iron. And what about that endless search for misplaced keys or glasses? It makes life harder. However, the other side of the coin is not a sure bet either. In psychology, this type of superhuman memory is called hypermnesia and researchers are still tossing up how to classify it—is it acceptable or abnormal?

> **"Poor memory is a drag. It limits your actions, makes you uncertain about yourself."**

This type of memory can bring a lot of negativity into people's lives. It's tough going through life remembering anything and everything. Every rude word spoken to you, your own silly mistakes, unpleasantness and hurt, tragic events, betrayal— you continue living through it, experiencing all those negative emotions. It's far better if your memory can eliminate these feelings over time, de-cluttering your mind like you would your physical space.

I want to share my personal experience of living with a person with a phenomenal memory. After being divorced for a number of years, I met a man who I fell in love with in my late fifties. Our relationship developed rapidly, and we got married very quickly.

He was a retired colonel with a loud voice and a plethora of knowledge on any possible subject. In the beginning, I admired it and was a respectful listener. His memory contained full chronology on any war on earth—precise dates, places, military operations, names of all the generals and their victories.

As if that was not enough, he remembered every name and surname of every soldier under his command for thirty years. He had stored all the addresses of all the people he had ever been in contact with. His stories were never-ending, filled with unnecessary, unrelated details. It was not fun—I needed an aspirin just to get through it. That was hypermnesia at its worst. To my view it is abnormal and—as you may have guessed—we are no longer together. It's best to have a memory with no blind spots and gaps but at the same time, it shouldn't hold on to useless, out-dated information. But is that easier said than done?

Mistakes and unpleasantness from your past should be removed. You don't need it, do you? Everything takes effort in life, including mental work. De-cluttering your memory is a job for the mind. Ideally, it should monitor the memory's content and periodically remove information that isn't needed anymore—just chuck it out!

You must have heard about a person who got amnesia, a total loss of memory. Maybe you've seen it in a movie. Physically, this person could be perfectly alright, except they remember nothing. Nothing at all—who they are, who the people around them are, where were they born and when. Then suddenly, under some physical or emotional shock, all their memories come back. Just like that, in the blink of an eye! This is undeniable proof that the memory is not ruined permanently. Our ability to read our memory—connecting to our memories and bringing them up to the surface—is what gets broken and subsequently restored.

So, when we want to remove an unwanted memory, we cannot actually just chuck it out, as it were. It stays in our brain somewhere, in a protected recycle bin with a sticker on it saying *access denied.* On a daily basis, an avalanche of new data is not just tossed in but sorted out by keywords. These pieces are arranged in such a way that allows us to instantaneously find and extract them on demand. For a better understanding of our memory, some people visualise it as if those bits of information are being put in to separate boxes and neatly placed on shelves in a strict, organised order. Certain memories are treasured by us—they must have a special place in close proximity so that we can relive them again whenever we want.

As Haruki Murakami said in his book *Kafka on the Shore,* "No matter how much time passes, no matter what takes place in the interim, there are some things we can never assign to oblivion, memories we can never rub away. They remain with us forever."

Unlike those hypermnesiacs, we mere mortals are often concerned with our memory. We all wish we had a better memory, don't we? Fortunately, for those who are prepared to work on its improvement, a large arsenal of techniques and methods are available to us. You will find a few useful training exercises under *System of Actions* in *Memory and Mnemonic Training.* The guiding principle is the same for all our natural abilities—use it or lose it.

Trust Your Memory

Many of us doubt our memory but the less we trust it, the less we rely on it. The less we rely on it, the less we use it and the less we use it, the less it works. The less it works, the less we trust it—and so the vicious cycle continues.

What if I told you that it is possible to change and improve your memory regardless of your age? It is true! For many of us, it is possible and achievable. Even if Mother Nature has not been generous and let you enter this world with a poor memory or attention span, you still have the ability to correct it and top it up with your own consistent efforts. As memory is a function of the brain, it can be developed and trained in the same way as any other function. We only differ by how fast or efficiently we are able to memorise things. Just follow these principles when you consider your own memory and the work you could do to improve it.

- All people have the memory.

- The memory is a function of the brain.

- Brain activity and function can be trained similarly to other organs.

- The more your memory works the stronger it becomes.

- The more things you memorise the easier it will be to memorise more.

We can make a fair comparison between memory and muscle. As our muscles can be trained, so can our memory. There are no good or bad muscles. With memory, it is a bit more complex, but the principle remains the same. Whatever you want to improve in life, you must invest time and effort. The memory includes three elements: memorising, retaining and recovery. Unfortunately, it is not in our power to organise a retaining process for storing and recovering information. Therefore, the only thing we can improve is the process of memorising. The stronger our desire to memorise something, the stronger our motivation is for keeping it on the surface of our memory. I want to share an incredible example of how strong motivation supports memorising, not just for us humans, but also for fish, especially when hunger is a motivator.

Research from Keio University, Tokyo revealed that fish can tell the difference between Stravinsky and Bach. Experiments revealed that the fish could learn and memorise the difference between the two composers through training with food. Hearing a Stravinsky piece, the fish rushed to their feeder but stayed impartial to magnificent Bach, as no food was available with his music. If fish can do it, so can you!

> **"When people complain about their memory loss, what is actually lost or broken is the ability to recall memories."**

When people complain about their memory loss, what is actually lost or broken is the ability to recall memories. It has been proven that memories never disappear from our brain and, in fact, it is the search mechanism that is the culprit. As we discussed earlier, there have been many cases recorded of individuals recovering memories after suffering from amnesia for many years. This happens when people experience an acute shock, either psychological or physical, like being struck by lightning.

As with anything else, memory training could significantly improve the ability to memorise, even in much older people. A correlation has been found between improved memorising and a heightened ability to recall things from the past. The more often you make your mental mechanisms register and reproduce things that you wish to memorise, the easier it becomes. Repetition is the key to any kind of training, including the memory.

Developing a strong memory can help us to memorise all the things that are important to us, large and small. It is different from hypermnesia in the sense that it can be developed through training. The art of developing a fantastic memory is called mnemonics and it has always attracted and fascinated people. In essence, mnemonics is a system based on a pattern of letters, ideas, or associations, which assists in remembering information.

It is an ancient technique developed by Giordano Bruno in the sixteenth century. You may remember him as the monk burned alive by the Roman Inquisition for heresy. However, in his time, Giordano was incredibly popular as a mnemonics guru, accepted by European royals and other dignitaries. King Henry III and his court, as well as other nobilities, loved learning about mnemonics, using it to entertain themselves and their distinguished guests.

Mnemonics teaches special skills on how to easily remember information with no logical connection between sequences of words, numbers, images or letters. Therefore, mnemonics is a tool to help remember facts or a large amount of information. It can be a song, rhyme, acronym, image or phrase to help remember a list of facts in a certain order. You find mnemonics training exercises in the third section, *System of Actions.*

SYSTEM OF GOALS

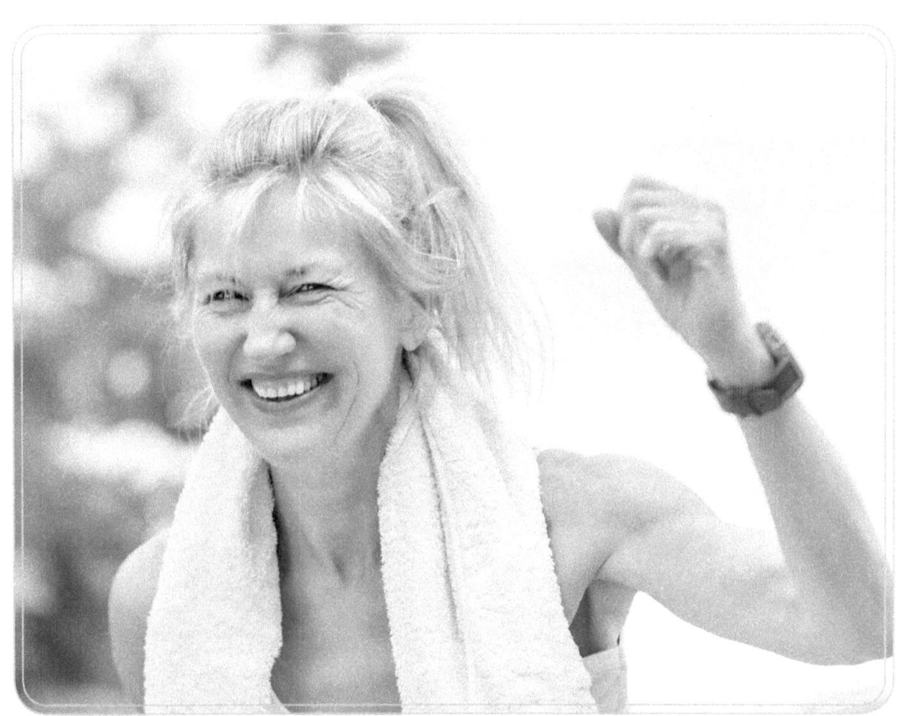

How to be S.M.A.R.T.

Goals are the last link in the chain—they start as a dream and become a desire. The desire then becomes stronger as it morphs into a more detailed picture. Then, by working on it, our mind transforms it into a goal. The goal must have characteristics or features that make it practical and achievable. These characteristics are well researched and established. This SMART formula is widely used by professionals working with people and stands for:

S — Specific

M — Measurable

A — Attainable

R — Relevant

T — Timely

SPECIFIC: This is when you need to ask yourself, "What exactly do I want to achieve?" The more specific your goal, the better

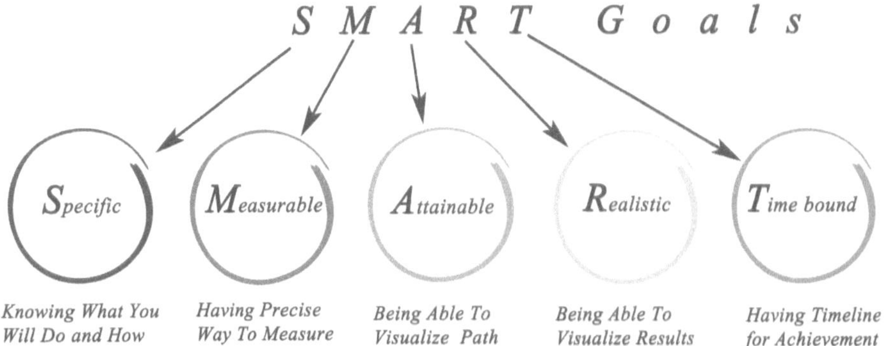

your chances of achieving it. When planning out your goal, try to answer the five 'W' questions:

- What do I want to accomplish?

- Why is this goal important?

- Who is involved?

- Where will I achieve this?

- Which resources or limits are involved?

> **"You are never too young to set goals for your longevity."**
> — Natsha Lukin

MEASURABLE: It's important to have measurable goals so you can track your progress and stay engaged. Being able to measure your progress helps you to stay focused, achieve your "by when" goals and feel the excitement of moving closer to the finish line.

ATTAINABLE: Is the goal you want attainable? You need to think about the effort, time and any other costs, and then assess any other commitments in your life. If you don't have the time, money or ability to reach your goal you'll probably be disappointed. That doesn't mean that you can't create a goal that seems impossible and make it happen by smart planning.

RELEVANT: Is your goal relevant to you? Do you really want to run a Fortune 500 company, be famous, have four children, get a puppy? You need to decide if it's what you really want and if you have what it takes. If you don't have all the skills required, you can invest in training. If you don't have certain resources available to you, you can always find a way to get them.

The big question is: why do you want to reach this goal? What is the intention behind the goal and will it actually provide you with what you desire?

TIMELY: As the saying goes, "Time is money!" It's important you make a plan of everything you do. We all know that a deadline is what makes most people take action. One thing to keep in mind is that your timeline needs to be realistic and flexible. Being too strict on the timing aspect of your goal can have a contradictory effect, turning the journey into a nightmarish race against time, which is not how you want to achieve anything.

Focus: How Your Dream Becomes a Goal

One more thing that could be included in the S.M.A.R.T. formula is 'focus'. You have set your goal and now it's time to work on the execution. There is a danger in changing your mind, and I am not talking about adjusting certain things along the way. What I mean is a loss of focus, listening to other peoples' opinions and doubting yourself.

Recently, I watched an animal documentary on TV. A leopard was preparing to jump on its prey. It was a mesmerising scene. The leopard was like a single, contracted muscle. Its gaze did not leave its victim for a second. Its tail quivered, revealing the power of its concentration. Ready, set, go—complete focus on the task.

Now, imagine if the leopard started thinking the way we sometimes do.

- "Will I be able to cover the distance in one jump?"
- "What if I fail to catch my prey?"

➔ "What will other leopards think about me?"

➔ "Maybe I should wait…?"

Recognisable? That is exactly how we allow ourselves to think, which prevents us from taking some of our best chances. Although it is not included in the formula, focus is equally important. Of course, the leopard in the documentary performed spectacularly. So, keep focused. Don't deviate or hesitate once your decision is made. Trust yourself.

A really huge, ambitious goal can seem insurmountable until it is broken down into smaller chunks. I remember a story from 15 years ago. I had a neighbour that became a good friend. Her name was Lara and she decided one day that she wanted a sea change. Lara was a reflexologist and masseuse in her early fifties, with eighteen-year-old twin sons.

The idea totally engulfed her. She talked about it all the time but was hesitant. These conversations went on for over a year. Then someone invited her to participate in a workshop in Byron Bay, an exclusive spot for all kinds of alternative people, from healers to clairvoyants, tattoo artists and surfers. As expected, Lara fell in love with the place. Her dream began to grow contours and gradually became a goal. She bought a special notebook and painstakingly described her dream.

"A really huge, ambitious goal can seem insurmountable until it is broken down into smaller chunks."

To work on a goal of such magnitude, Lara decided to break down her dream into smaller, more manageable chunks. I was her sounding board. She checked in with me about how she was doing, checking she was on the right track. Under each section, she listed every task that she needed to achieve and by when. This dream had now become a S.M.A.R.T. goal. She had asked herself all the right questions and she was taking action.

I was impressed with how she was going about everything. She was following her plan without haste, step-by-step, staying focused on her goal. I found her approach motivational. With each step, I watched her become more inspired and confident. We still keep in touch and I've heard Lara is popular as a healer and alternative therapist.

Having a dream that becomes a goal is essential to our longevity. In a way, it creates a purpose for our lives. A person without a purpose is like a yacht without sails or an anchor.

In our younger years, it happens auto-matically—we grow, learn, study, work, get married, have kids, improve on our career, socialise with friends, co-workers, our kids' school friends' parents, etc. The purposes and goals are there all the time. Then, one sunny day, we retire and hear a chorus of friendly voices, congratulating us on our retirement, telling us how lucky we are now we can live the way we want, do whatever we want and enjoy our life.

> **"Now you live in a new reality that requires a different attitude and the re-evaluation of your life purpose and goals."**

That is when a turbulent period of your life starts. It could have taken a few years for the dust to settle down and a new chapter of your life to begin. In the course of my interaction with clients, I often come across people who are either uncertain about their desires or cannot even formulate them. Some have desires but, on examination, it turns out that those desires were actually suggested to them by other people, like parents, authorities, mass media or those friends who "know better".

In both cases, these desires have no chance of being fulfilled. The absence of desires or not having them fulfilled can be a road to depression, which affects a person's health and their life circumstances, pushing them into an unavoidable, downward spiral.

The type of depression that is most difficult to cure is known as "the crisis of desires", a sad diagnosis—if a person has no desires, it's like they have no desire for life.

The Pen is Mightier Than the Sword

Firstly, goals need to be put down on paper. A goal written down in full detail has much more chance of success than one held only in your mind. When we first try to describe our goals verbally we often stumble. That is why goal setting must be done with a pen in your hand. Remember, "The pen is mightier than the sword". When we write our goals down, it activates our subconscious, providing certainty and revealing new pathways to our goals. Secondly, a correctly set-up goal implies its positive intention. Therefore, it works to present a goal as an affirmation, meaning you talk about what you want, not about what you don't want.

When writing goals down, it is important to create them as positive statements, focusing on what you want rather than what you don't want. For example, instead of "I don't want to be fat anymore" say "I want to slim down to 65 kilograms". If the thoughts circling in your mind are "I don't want this", the best thing to do is ask yourself "what *do* I want?" This will also shift your energy and allow you to focus, which makes you feel great.

Thirdly, other words that don't work when creating goals are words that create resistance as they diminish the goal's value. I'll show you a simple demonstration with two sentences. Think about the sentence, "I need some rest and should go on holiday". How about something like, "I will rest one hour each day and I will go on a holiday once a year for ten days"?

You can really feel the difference when you read both of these out loud—the second one almost feels like you have achieved it already.

When we focus our attention on a goal with all our mental strength directed on it, then both our conscious and unconscious minds will deliver. That is how prayers work. When we say a prayer with the utmost concentration on our needs, wants and goals, our positive energy can materialise.

I wish to share my understanding of spirituality. I trust that a higher power exists, and we are all a part of it. There is too much proof, both on a planetary level and in our personal lives. In my view, the question is whether we recognise the power's existence or not. Everything else is a matter of terminology. We say things like "higher being", "God", "cosmic energy" or other symbolic names or images but, in essence, we speak about the same thing.

Why Some Vision Boards Work and Others Don't

When setting goals, working with images can be very helpful. Vision boards or desire cards are now very well utilised. However, it takes special skills and a lot of mind-power to reach your desired outcome. Allow me to explain why some vision boards

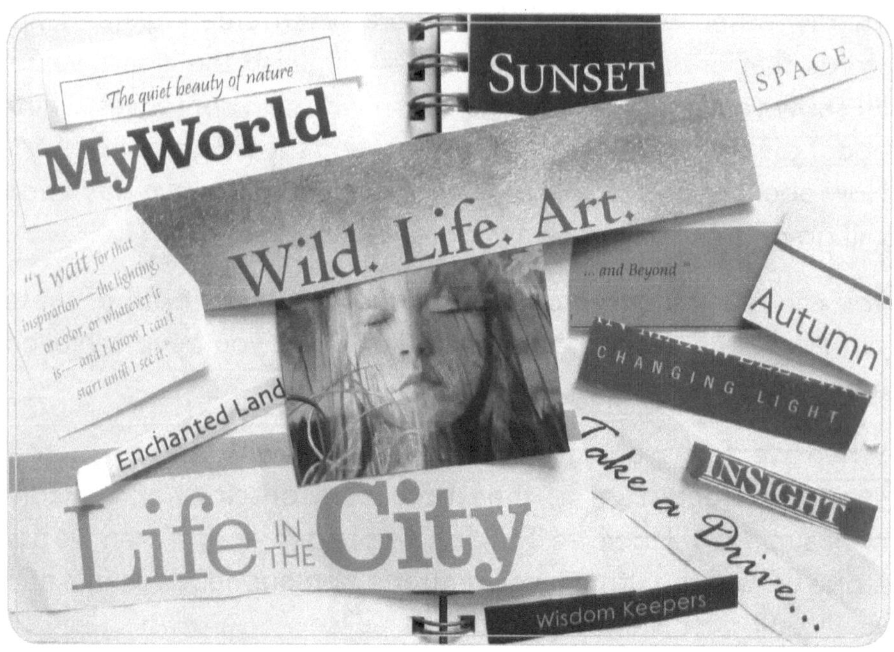

work, and others don't. Sometimes our desires don't fit into the S.M.A.R.T. formula because not all the points are applicable. In this case, a great tool to use may be a visual board. However, to present your desires in real images means to transfer those images into your mind. It works wonders.

The vision board plays the role of the programming device. It activates the universal law of attraction by observing the images and phrases you have chosen to manifest your dreams into reality. It is a combined work of imagination, visual perception and passion in your heart for the realisation of your desire. You also need to recognise that these processes are rituals that are beyond reasoning. Instead, they should be followed to the letter.

This is a real-life example of how it worked out for my friend Yvonne. She was 47 at the time, a divorcee, and set a goal to find her Mr Right. Gradually, she became addicted to introductory websites, spending all her spare time on them. I cannot tell you how many sites she was registered on—I lost count. First, Yvonne checked Australian sites, then moved to international ones. She was totally engrossed in these activities: talking on the phone or Skype, meeting men for coffee, etc.

All of this consumed an enormous amount of her time with no real gain. To cut it short, we decided to make her a vision board and she took it seriously. We didn't just pin pictures to it as so many people do.

It was a rigorous process of selecting pictures from magazines, brochures and even printing some from the internet. These were photos and drawings of wedding decorations, flowers, attractive men and couples doing things together—things that Yvonne wanted to do.

She talked to each image, absorbing them into her conscious mind, keeping them close to her mouth to warm them up with her breath. Then we made those images into collages. We placed some quotations on the board and a deadline for Yvonne's meeting with her destiny.

> **"The vision board plays the role of the programming device. It activates the universal law of attraction by observing the images and phrases you have chosen to manifest your dreams into reality."**

The board now looked like a work of art. Every morning and night, Yvonne continued talking to the images. The deadline arrived, and nothing had happened. We both felt deflated about it and arranged to meet for lunch at our favourite café in Malvern.

As soon as we entered, we saw him. All the tables were taken, and he was sitting by himself, no other seats available. He gestured to us as if inviting us to take a seat at his table. Yvonne and the man looked at each other—and the rest was history. When we talked about their meeting much later, Gerald confessed that he was passing through on the way to a different place, but something made him take a detour and step into that café.

What a wonderful example of how powerful a vision board can be if executed correctly. It became a direct request for the desired outcome and it worked. However, I know some people who have been disappointed with their vision boards and I know why. In spite of the procedure seemingly being done properly, they did not implant the images into their unconscious mind. They saw the pictures and collages as static, mental images, failing to imbue them with energy. So, they stayed as they were—just pictures.

Excuses and Other Calamities

Excuses, reasons and explanations hinder our best intentions and become blocks on the road towards our goals. We all have excuses for why we aren't doing something that we have planned to do. What if we didn't use excuses anymore? Getting clear on how our excuses work against our intentions and goals will help us to identify and deal with them.

Are our excuses and reasons helpful, supportive of our goals or useful in any other way? The answer is no. What matters is the result and *only* the result—nothing else. Let's see what is preventing us from achieving our goals so we can get the results we are striving for.

There are four major groups of obstacles. Do you ever come across the situation where you have set your goal and then immediately begin sabotaging it? Take me for instance, setting the goal to go for a walk every morning. A simple goal— specific, measurable, attainable. To avoid getting up early and going for a walk, I have

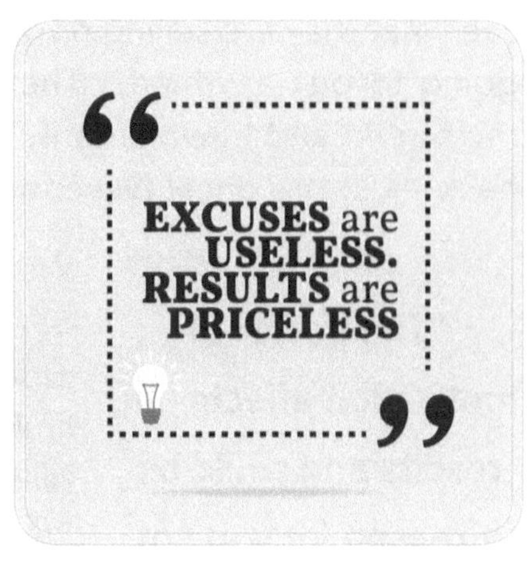

all sorts of excuses and I truly believe in them at that moment. It's too cold, too hot, too windy. I don't really feel like it this morning. I've got too much to do at home before work. I need more sleep, etc.

Some of those sound like legitimate excuses, but are they? We can call them reasons but that doesn't change the fact that, because of them, we haven't produced the results we wanted. The result is achieving your goal. Of course, things happen. God forbid, if you fell and broke your leg and it is now in plaster, that is a fully acceptable reason for not going for a walk, but we are looking at excuses that work against our goals and most of them don't hold any merit.

Another way we fool ourselves is to state what we are going to do rather than not do. I will put myself on display again. I have to confess, at one time, I was addicted to online shopping. Mostly clothing but other stuff as well. So, I set myself a goal— stop going online every day and no more internet purchases. My wardrobe was bursting with stuff and some of it I hadn't even worn. Now, let's see how I sabotaged my goal. My fingers automatically typed a web address of an online store. "I just want to see what they are selling now," I told myself. "Of course, I'm not going to buy anything." Then the loveliest dress appeared on my screen and I involuntarily clicked on it. "80% off? What the heck—just this once! Never again."

> **"The power of motivation affects our results and could be a reason for you not achieving your goal."**

We know that we often overestimate our capabilities. However, as we get older, we have to acknowledge our limitations, especially when we are talking about people of the so-called "third age". I don't want to discourage anyone from living life to the full. We just need to be realistic because there are still so many things we can do, explore and enjoy now when we have more free time on our hands. A great tool instilled in us by default is common sense. We might have to limit our physical exertion, but our life experience and knowledge can help us to find the balance between what we want to do and what we actually *can do*. By acting wisely, we can still get a lot of fun and enjoyment without taking too much risk.

Those who like comfort usually set goals that don't require too much effort or stress. Others are not afraid of effort. Their priority is to go beyond a habitual way of life and do something different and exciting. However, to set such a goal we have to evaluate our resources and means for achieving it. There is no single, correct solution for the magnitude of the goal. Only you personally know what is right for you. Just choose wisely.

The power of motivation affects our results and could be a reason for you not achieving your goal. We have to keep in mind that both a lack of motivation and excess of motivation equally hinder the process. This was established in 1908 by two scientists, Robert Yerkes and John Dodson, and became known as "Yerkes Dodson Law". They carried out research on how the power of motivation affects the results of activities depending on the level of difficulty of the task. Experiments were conducted on rats, chickens, cats and humans.

The scientists came up with the conclusion that if the motivation was not strong enough, the tasks would not be complete. However, excessive strong motivation also impacted their success as it led to unnecessary bustling and agitation that ruined their goal. So, other questions to ask yourself when setting goals are:

- "Do I need to break my goal down into smaller more manageable steps?"

- "When shall I start and when do I want to achieve my goal by?"

- "How will I monitor and manage my goal?"

Decide on the process of measuring steps and any interim results, and how you will identify if your goal has been achieved. In his wonderful book *Excuses Begone*, Dr Wayne Dyer taught us about controlling our thoughts. He says to "think about what we are thinking about". This can be applied to how we think about our goals and where our excuses are coming from.

Dr Dyer believed that "our excuses come from operating from the limited space of our ego, and often times we have no indisputable evidence that our excuses hold any merit". When we take control of our mind then we master the art of setting our goals and making viable plans. Doing so can bring more peace and enjoyment. How often do we hear excuses like "as soon as the weather gets better…" or "…when I sort out my paperwork, I will"?

However, if life is postponed until later, that later just might not happen. What could help a person to get out of the trap of endless excuses and reasons, and start living today, right now? The simplest way is: act. That's right, just act. Not spending too much time on reasoning, or discussing colourful plans, goals and desires with friends—start taking action instead.

Dealing with Problems

It's rare not to encounter problems when we work on our goals. How can we deal with unexpected obstacles, various delays or changes of circumstances? There is often a pattern in our reactions to our problems. First of all, we see our problems as if we are looking through a magnifying glass. It is almost inevitable that they seem far larger and important to us than they are. That is human nature—I look at my problem and it spreads to the horizon, covering such a huge space that it looks like there is no way out.

Therefore, we need to step back and gain a different perspective. A great way to do this is to imagine that this is someone else's problem. It will shrink in front of your eyes immediately. Then you begin reasoning about how that person is supposed to cope. You start thinking about the advice you could offer. This is actually the first step to looking at your own solution.

The Logic Mind Assumes, While the Subconscious Mind Knows

To live life being guided by logic only is not productive. Seeking logical explanation for everything around us and making decisions strictly based on logic only results in more fear and disappointment. Logic is often blocking our centre of free will. With time, usually at about the age of 45, we begin to experience a feeling that we are trapped. That is the age of divorce, plans for sea or tree changes, changing jobs, etc. Our soul is looking for a way out of logic's tight embrace.

If we rely only on logic, we are not questioning our intuition and imagination. The best recipe is to check our logical actions against our intuition. Our "inner whisper" is rarely loud and it would be so valuable to develop a habit to listen to it before making our final decision. The whole thing can be explained in simple words—the logic mind assumes, while the subconscious mind knows.

Speaking of goals, logic dictates how to follow rules, how to play it safe and how not to make mistakes. It is useful to a certain degree and keeps us in our comfort zone. However, brilliant discoveries and fantastic results are never achieved if we obediently stay inside our boundaries. Logic often prevents us from taking bold, courageous and challenging steps. Therefore, it is often what's really behind our excuses. And you know what? Sometimes, just not giving the problem too much of your attention can really make a difference.

The Secret of Rocambole

Between 1857 and 1870 the first superhero and adventurer, Rocambole, a French fictional character, kept Europe captivated. A chain of novels was published in newspapers and became a highly popular serial read. A few times, the author and the publisher tried to kill Rocambole off but the public, in indignation, demanded his return. Not only was he incarcerated in prison, his face burned by acid and his body disfigured, he was

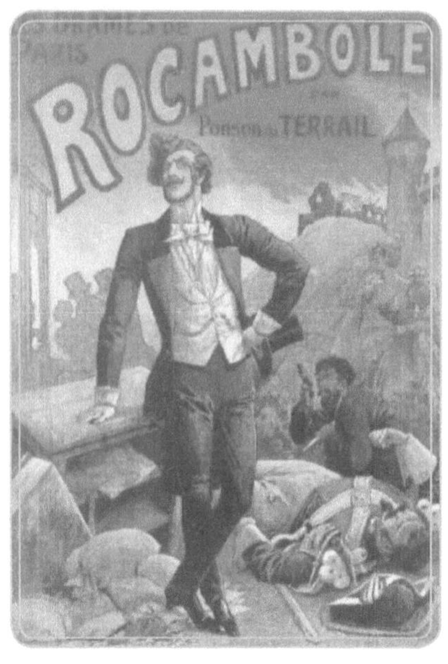

subjected to torture and other horrible, unfortunate events. However, Rocambole reappeared from the ashes every time and continued to entertain the public.

Maxim Gorky wrote, "Rocambole taught me to be resilient and not to succumb to the power of circumstances". However, one day, as the story goes, it was a heated argument that ensued after the author asked for a pay rise that finally saw Rocambole killed off for good. He was chained up, locked in an iron box, taken by boat to the middle of the ocean and chucked overboard. Now, Rocambole rests at the bottom of the sea.

This triggered a huge public outcry. The newspaper began rapidly losing subscribers and the publisher called on other writers, asking them to bring the character back to life. They all scratched their heads—no one could figure out a way of saving him. It just didn't seem plausible. As the newspaper's circulation hit rock-bottom, the publisher had no other option but to offer a huge financial reward to the original author. The very next week, an ecstatic public queued for the paper to read the next part of Rocambole's adventure. It started with, "Free again, Rocambole strolled along Les Champs-Élysées in Paris..."

> **"Sometimes, by some strange ways in life, everything is adjusted by itself". — Max Frey**

Nobody cared how the hero had managed to save himself. He had done it and that was what mattered. The question of *how* could be left open. Who really cared? Rocambole was alive and kicking and the public was happy to have him back.

What is the lesson here? Sometimes, by simply ignoring the problem, it dissipates by itself. Not always and not often, but it happens. Perhaps, if we focus too much on a problem, it could become more important that it deserves to be.

How to Go from Knowing What to Do … to Actually Doing It

When people say 'procrastination is laziness' I tend to disagree. Procrastinators are often very busy people. They are doing a lot—to avoid what they *should* be doing as a matter of priority.

Why do they do it? One of the possible explanations is that the task at hand is daunting because of its size or having too many aspects to it. Maybe they don't have enough clarity on where to start or a lack of vision for the expected outcome. Perhaps it simply requires too much effort.

If a task is overwhelming, people will deploy a variety of excuses and mental tricks to subconsciously avoid taking even the first step in executing it.

They suddenly find things to do like washing the dishes, making a phone call to an old friend, remembering to write a letter to their internet provider, sending an email to their book club—and the list goes on.

> "Procrastination is the thief of time."
> — Edward Young.

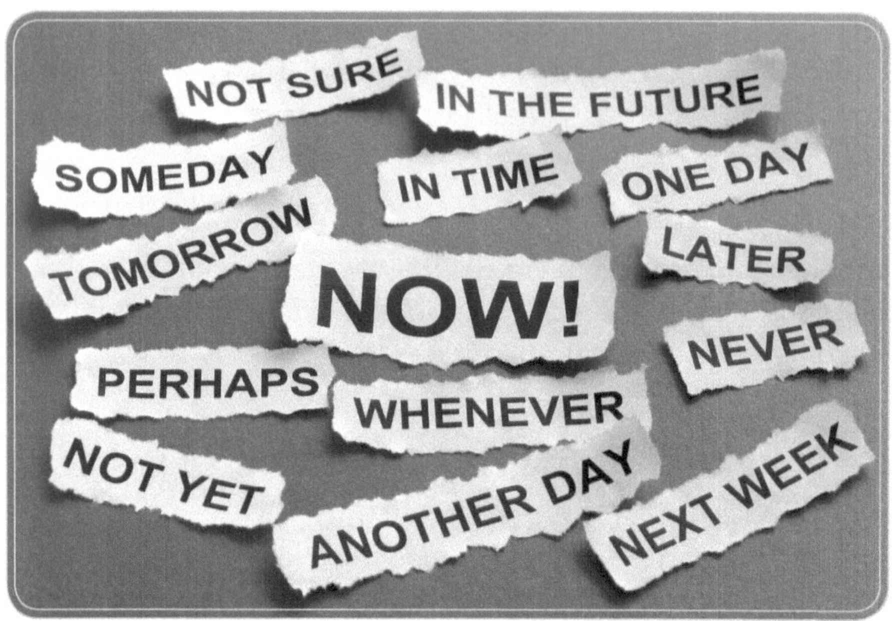

If it becomes a regular pattern in your behaviour, it becomes a habit. Then, gradually, this can become a severe problem leading to disappointment in yourself, lingering stress and depression. Without fulfilling obligations, the procrastinator begins to feel guilty, loses faith in themselves and develops a serious, psychological disorder.

According to Noah St John, there are three reasons why procrastination is the thief of time:

1. Time never stops or slows down—it's always moving.

2. Once it's gone, it's gone forever.

3. Therefore, time is the one resource that can never be replaced.

If you spend money, you can always get it back. If you expend energy, you can usually replenish it. But all of Bill Gates' billions can't buy one minute of yesterday.

The main culprit for procrastination is a lack of desire, multiplied by laziness and a lack of willpower or a lack of interest. In addition, another reason for procrastination is an inability to prioritise.

Someone who found a solution for the treatment of procrastination was Dwight Eisenhower, the 34th President of the United States, serving two terms from 1953 to 1961. Before becoming president, Eisenhower was a five-star general in the United States Army and the Supreme Commander of the Allied Forces in Europe during World War II. This is a remarkable story confirming that a great mind is always a great mind.

So, what happened when he was elected the President of the United States? In the beginning, he was overwhelmed by the avalanche of matters and issues requiring his attention. One day, Eisenhower sat down and scrupulously jotted down everything he had to do. It was such a long list that it made him shiver. To cope with it, Eisenhower placed himself in a familiar situation. He imagined that this was not a list of presidential tasks, but the enemy army.

He began to study his enemy and discovered that it was not that scary. He discovered that all his tasks were subjects of differing importance. He began seeing a clearer picture and found that all his matters could be divided into four categories:

1. Urgent and important (tasks you will do immediately).

2. Important, but not urgent (tasks you will schedule to do later).

3. Urgent, but not important (tasks you will delegate to someone else).

4. Neither urgent nor important (tasks that you will eliminate).

What he created was later named the "Eisenhower Matrix", or "Eisenhower Box". The great thing was that the Eisenhower Matrix provided a clear framework for making decisions. Like anything in life, consistency is the hard part. Here is an example of how it might look.

- Take a sheet of paper and make your to-do list.

- For each task, assign a status of importance.

- Transfer your tasks into the Matrix's squares in accordance with their status.

Do first	Do later
Urgent & Important Important tasks that require immediate attention.	**Not Urgent & Important** Important tasks that don't require immediate action.
Delegate	**Eliminate**
Urgent & Not Important Activities that require immediate action, but do not contribute to our goals.	**Not Urgent & Not Important** Tasks that are neither important nor urgent.

When finished, look at the box in the top-left, "Urgent and Important". These are the tasks you need to start without delay. Pick the top task and go for it. That is what will help you to beat procrastination. Executing your first task will make you feel better about yourself. You'll need to draw a new matrix every day for 30 days. Every day, you'll fill all four boxes with tasks according to their status. This will allow you to effectively manage your time.

After finishing his presidency, Eisenhower continued as a popular speaker. Eisenhower once asked a large audience how many of them were using his Matrix. Many hands went up. Then he asked how many of them emptied that top-left corner box. There was only one person with his hand up—the current vice president. Eisenhower said, "The one who manages his time so perfectly will be able to manage anything—not just the nation but the universe itself."

Many of us know that feeling of resistance in making the first step and how hard it can be to say to ourselves, "Just *do* it!" However, even science supports the idea of getting started, irrespective of whether you are ready or not. The laws of physics state that it is easier to keep going than get going, so start the task, even before you feel motivated to do it.

Here's some advice from famous business coach Shamim Rafeek: "Practice creative procrastination. Since we can't do everything, we must learn to deliberately put off those tasks that are of low value so that we have enough time to do the few things that really count."

Other Tips for Doing Things

- → "Bribe yourself," says Prof Piers Steel, author of *The Procrastination Equation*.

- → Procrastinators know how to do 40 minutes' work in 7 hours and how to do 7 hours' work in 40 minutes.

- → "Break it down," says Prof Joe Ferarri, author of *Still Procrastinating? The No Regrets Guide to Getting It Done.*

- → "Procrastinators struggle to see the wood for the trees; I say cut down one tree. If that's too much, cut down one branch. If that's too much cut me some leaves. Just do it!"

Living through our golden years, we don't have a lot of time to waste. We still have time to live and enjoy our life, but we need to live our quality time with gusto, not wasting it doing unimportant tasks and feeling guilty for not doing what is really important. Therefore, I suggest we stop procrastinating. Consider it as though we have been granted additional time to spend more wisely.

SYSTEM OF ACTIONS

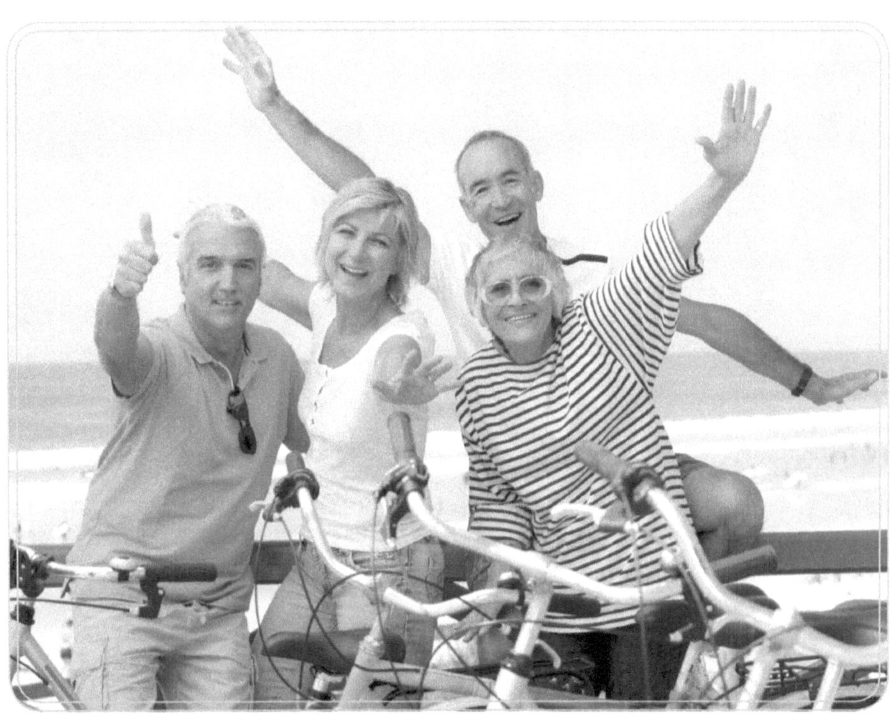

The Secret of Looking Young

For some people, the concept of "looking younger" is limited by the look of the skin on their face. With tons of skincare products screaming at us from every screen and paper, we are bound to believe that smooth and radiant skin is the only definition of looking younger.

I have no objection to improving your skin texture and colour using creams, lotions, moisturisers, concealers, foams, etc. as well as cosmetic procedures using radio frequencies and electrophoresis. Then the heavy artillery follows—fillers, Botox, and plastic surgery. I'm okay with all of that too. But is it all worth it? How can this person who claims to "look younger" be accurately assessed on their claim?

Let's start with what we can see from a distance. First, you would see their movements, their gait. If they walk hunched, shuffling their legs, no amount of cream on their face will win them any points for looking younger over unattractive, heavy or small, fussy footsteps. Then their gestures, the plasticity of their hands, how their head is "sitting" on their neck and how they turn it. Also, their posture—is their head in a forward position with rolled shoulders?

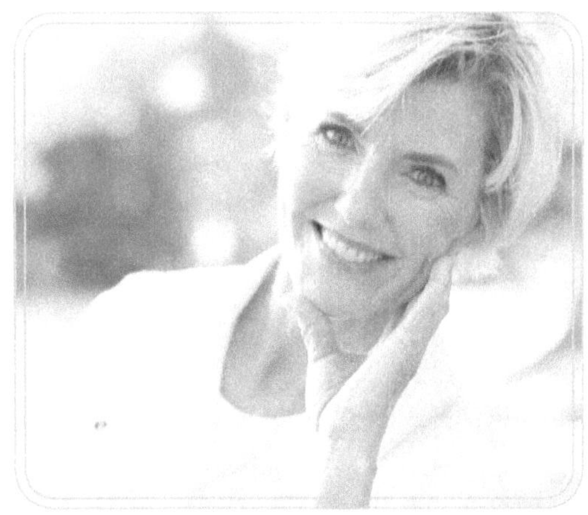

These movements unmistakably reveal the difference between young and old. Ask a friend to take a video of you when you are moving and see for yourself how others see you. Then decide what should be improved.

The next thing asking for attention is your figure. This is not necessarily about being slim. You can have lots of curves and still look extremely attractive if you know how to present your body and what to wear.

And now we look at the face. Who would look younger? Imagine a face with smooth skin stretched from ear to ear without a single line, but with lacklustre, dull eyes, and practically no expression. In comparison, a face with bright, engaging eyes, a natural smile and a few lines and creases. Which one is more appealing?

Those smooth, soulless faces look like they all came out of the same mould. Their skin does not really conceal their age. We still see it, regardless of the quality of cosmetics. The ones with shiny eyes convey the younger feel. Again, the age could be easily guessed, but their sincere nature shines through, unconstrained by fillers or Botox. The tell-tale signs are your smile and laugh. A sincere, open smile reflected in your eyes and unconstrained laughter conveys a feeling of youth.

Clear Vision

Therefore, to make a face look "younger", I would put an emphasis on caring for your eyes. One of the most successful eye training programs is The Bates Method and it has been used since early last century. It is also known as "Clear Vision". By doing Dr Bates' exercises regularly, you can preserve and recover the clarity of your eyes.

Dr William H. Bates worked as an orthodox ophthalmologist in New York City and was considered an authority by members of his profession throughout many decades. His regime is still in widespread use today, although not without some controversy. The Bates method is used for short sight, long sight, astigmatism, presbyopia, squints, "lazy" eyes and even structural diseases such as macular degeneration. Bates found that all could benefit from learning to relax the eyes and mind.

> **"All day long, use your eyes right. You have just as much time to use your eyes right as you have to use them wrong." — Dr Bates**

Dr Bates maintained that most visual problems are due to a misuse of the visual system. He observed the habits of normal-sighted people and the characteristics of normal vision and devised ways to help people with abnormal sight relearn how to use their eyes naturally. As far back as 1922, Bates recommended: "All day long, use your eyes right. You have just as much time to use your eyes right as you have to use them wrong. It is easier and more comfortable to have perfect sight than to have imperfect sight."

The Bates Method can help almost anyone improve and often completely restore their vision. It works in most cases. Dr Bates' special eye exercises can free you from such conditions as short-sightedness, far-sightedness, squints, cataracts and glaucoma.

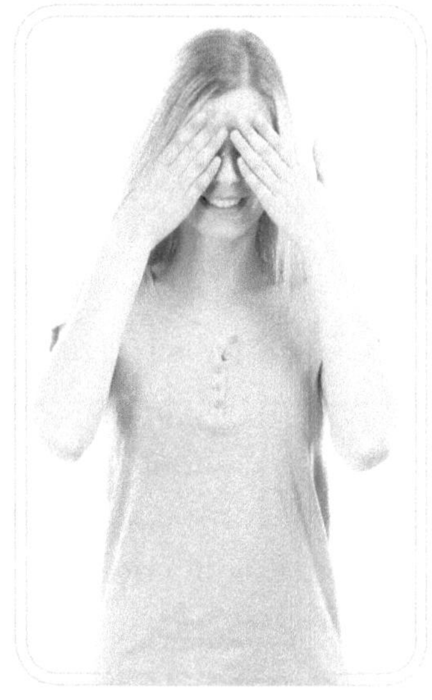

If you are interested, you can find many sources online or you can find his books in the library. Just by doing Bates' "Clear Vision" exercises, you will experience noticeable improvements in your eyesight.

In a nutshell, for a younger-looking face, we need bright eyes, a healthy smile and a natural facial expression.

Say Goodbye to Lines and Sagging Skin

The skin on your face is very delicate. Unfortunately, most of us have been subjected to a host of creams and lotions that are overly expensive and filled with chemicals that don't often bring the desired results. What if I told you there is a fantastic substance for healing many facial skin problems without any side effects that costs you next-to-nothing?

It is a mixture of two basic ingredients—coconut oil and bicarbonate of soda. Both are known for their antiseptic and anti-inflammatory properties. Bicarbonate of soda has a pH-balancing effect on your skin and can be used for acne treatment as well as teeth-whitening and can also be used as a deodorant. Coconut oil is full of nutrients and cleans and hydrates the skin. These two ingredients mix into a paste that can be used instead of soap or various lotions.

In a small bowl mix together one tablespoon of bicarbonate of soda with two tablespoons of coconut oil. Apply the paste to your face in a circular motion. Leave on for ten minutes. Then rinse it off with warm water. Coconut oil is deeply hydrating for the skin, so you won't need a moisturiser afterwards. These ingredients are easy to find, natural and cheap. Start using this paste and you will be very happy with your clean and radiant skin.

Butter mask for the face

The combination of butter and semolina is life-giving indeed. Semolina contains starch, vegetable protein and fibre, which is an invaluable food for the skin. Even using this mask once you will see an immediate, fantastic effect. Of course, it's better to do it as an extended course of treatment and repeat the procedure daily for at least a week.

Ingredients:

- 1 teaspoon of butter.

- 1/2 teaspoon of semolina.

How to apply:

- It's very important to use fresh and high-quality, unsalted butter with no less than 80% fat content. Melt the butter and mix it with the semolina.

- Apply to clean skin and leave for 15 minutes. Apply it quickly after mixing—semolina absorbs liquid fast and swells.

- Rinse the mask with warm water first, then with cold.

Flax seeds for a facelift

A simple mask made from flax seeds is surprisingly effective. You will forget about Botox and other expensive salon procedures if you start doing the following.

In the morning, prepare the tightening substance for the facelift that you will use in the evening. Pour a cup of boiling water over 1 teaspoon of flax seeds, mix well, cover with a tissue and leave to infuse.

In the evening:

- Wash your face.

- Lay down—the mask must be done lying down.

- Take the flax seed infusion and a sponge.

- Soak the sponge in the solution and apply it to your face, neck and décolletage.

- Let it dry.

- Apply another layer and let it dry.

- Repeat at least six times.

- Wash it off with clean water.

- **Enjoy the results.**

Facial Expressions

We have 43 muscles in our face—it takes each one of those 43 muscles to frown and only 17-26 to smile. Our facial expressions send a lot of information that is then received, understood and interpreted by others. They can reveal our emotional state, our feelings and reactions, our personality, mood, health status and even our biological age.

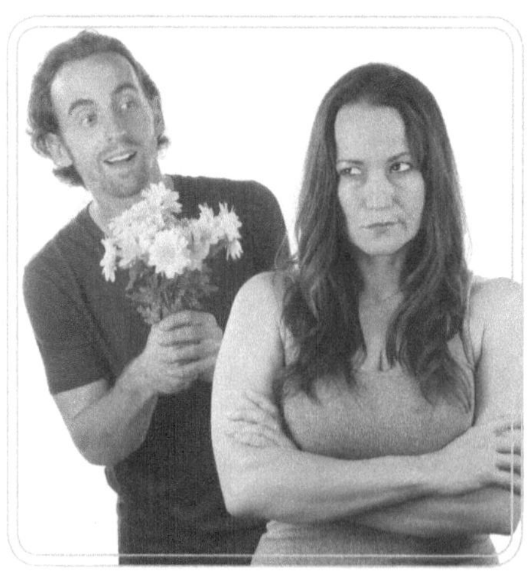

In our culture, we place great attention on exercise. Those 43 facial muscles can also be exercised with fantastic results. They can keep the face uplifted, reduce sagging, lines and creases. This also applies to the neck. The ligaments and muscles of your neck support your head and enable your range of motion. Those muscles and ligaments can also benefit from special exercises. One of these benefits could be a longer, straighter neck. The neck is a clear indicator for revealing a person's age, more so than any other feature.

So, if we want to get a quick result for a younger look, I recommend these three simple exercises for your neck. Soon, people will compliment you on looking refreshed and brighter, all thanks to these neck exercises.

Have you heard of the famous model, Carmen Del Orefice? She is an 86-year-old fashion icon preserving her elegance and style into her advanced years, setting a striking example of beauty beyond longevity. The following exercises are a part of her daily routine that we can all follow.

Warm-Up

- Tilt your head forward and back.

- Turn your head left and right.

- Tilt your head towards your left shoulder, then to the right shoulder.

- No sharp movements, do it smoothly. Keep your spine straight.

EXERCISE 1

First thing in the morning, lay down on your bed or couch in such a way that your head is hanging down. Lift your head trying to touch your chest with your chin.

EXERCISE 2

Sit up straight and put both fists under your chin. Now try to push your chin down while your fists resist this movement. Feel your neck muscles strain. Repeat five to seven times, three times a day. Rumour has it that this exercise was specifically developed for the ballet star Anna Pavlova and that Maya Plisetskaya, another great ballet dancer, also loved it.

EXERCISE 3

This one consists of three steps:

- Move your lower jaw forward as far as you can.

- Staying in that position, move your whole head forward. Then pull your shoulders back until your shoulder blades touch each other.

- Make a pout with your lips.

Repeat a few times. Then relax your head and neck.

> **"The internal smile is sincere, emanating from the whole body, including all organs, glands, muscles, bones and the nervous system."**

In her book, Carmen Del Orefice tells the story of how she discovered these exercises:

"One day, Diana Vreeland (a legendary editor of *Harper's Bazaar*) told me, 'I wish you could have a photo session in Paris with Richard Avedon, but your neck, Carmen, is not long enough. He might not like it.' Diana told me that I had to imagine that my neck was long and to practice some special exercises. We agreed to meet back at her office in a week's time to see if it worked for me. What can I say? I went to Paris..."

The Mona Lisa Smile

The internal smile, also known as The Mona Lisa Smile, is a very powerful practice of healing, originating from ancient China. Many people spend their lives experiencing anger, sadness, depression, fear, anxiety and other kinds of negative energy. These energies cause chronic illness and drain our vitality. 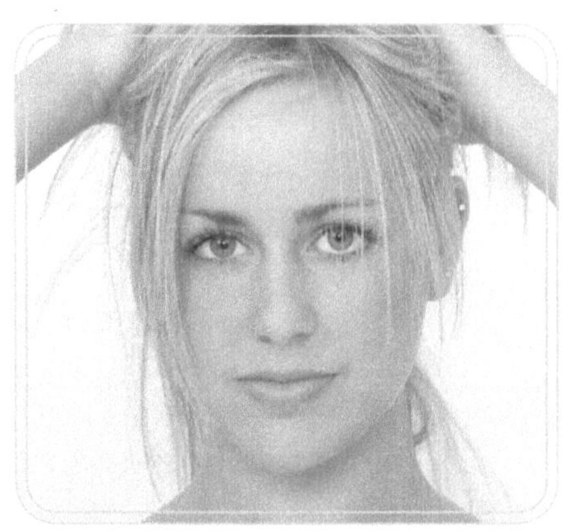 The internal smile is sincere, emanating from the whole body, including all organs, glands, muscles, bones and the nervous system. It produces high-quality energy that can heal and eventually transform itself into even higher quality energy.

A sincere smile sends a loving energy that has the power to heal and transform. Remember a time when you were upset or physically ill; someone—perhaps even a stranger—smiled sincerely and suddenly, you felt better. The internal smile directs loving energy into our organs and glands, which is necessary for healing and good life. The internal smile is the best medicine for neutralising any kind of stress.

11 Steps to Practicing the Inner Smile

1. Sit comfortably and keep your spine in an upright position—relax.

2. Take a couple of slow, deep breaths, noticing how your abdomen rises and relax with each breath.

3. Rest the tip of your tongue gently on the roof of your mouth.

4. Smile gently, allowing your lips to feel full and smooth as they spread to the side and lift just slightly.

5. Now bring your attention to the space between your eyebrows—your "third eye". Focus on this centre and feel gentle vibrations there.

6. Bring your attention now to the centre of your brain. This is a place referred to in Taoism as the "crystal palace". Feel the energy gathering in the middle of your head.

7. Allow this energy to flow forward into your eyes. Feel your eyes "smiling".

8. Now, direct the energy of your smiling eyes back and down into someplace in your body where you need healing, where you've recently had an injury or illness.

9. Continue to smile into that place within your body and let it absorb this energy like a sponge soaking up nourishing water.

10. When this feels complete, direct your inner smile into your solar plexus.

11. Release the tip of your tongue from the roof of your mouth and let the smile go.

When your energy grows, you will become more flexible and adaptable. You will know what you want in life and how to achieve it.

Fitness for Health and Enjoyment

To run or not to run—that is the question. Presently, we are in the middle of a controversial discussion regarding how much physical exertion is good for you. The division between people promoting heavy physicality to stay healthy, and those who call us back to relax on the couch, is growing wider. At both sides of the argument, we see professional people—doctors, sports physicians and physiotherapists as well as trainers and athletes.

Fitness gurus and their supporters are absolutely convinced that, to stay healthy and prolong youthfulness one should run a few kilometres in the morning, take part in weekend marathons, work out with weights and dumbbells in a gym, sweating profusely, and consider fitness to be the key to a happy and long life. However, in the last decade, we have heard different voices warning of the danger of overexertion.

William Campbell Douglass II, an American doctor, alternative medicine promoter and the self-termed "conscience of modern medicine" addressed his patients in his direct and sarcastic manner:

> "Even though everyone else is giving up coffee, alcohol, meat, eggs, fatty foods, sunshine and all things that make life liveable, and even though they're exer-cising like maniacs, sweating like horses and then scold *you* for not joining them, please don't submit to this self-denial because it's just *junk medicine*. It may look like the real thing, but when you see what it actually does to you, you'll be appalled".

"If you love going to the gym and working out, that is your choice. If you hate going to gym, if you're looking for an excuse not to go, if you are tired and miserable afterwards, that means you are making the wrong choice."

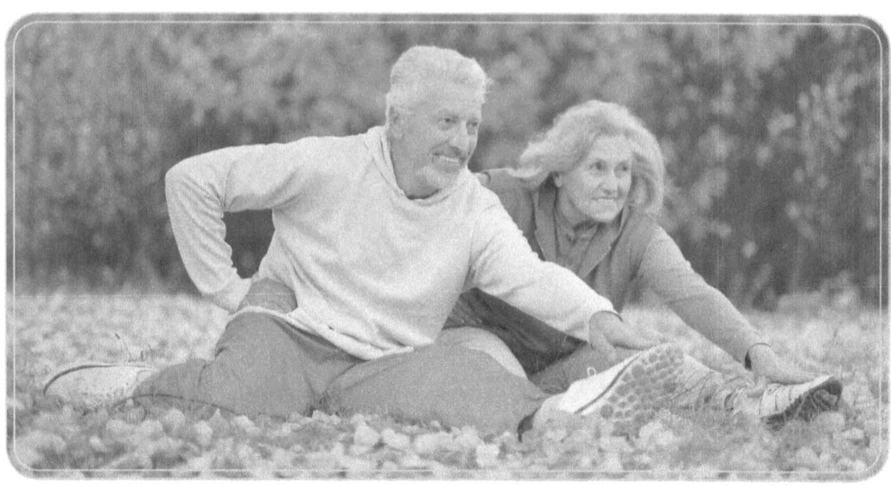

That is one very strong opinion, but the beauty of medicine is that there is no concept, theory or recommendation that one would not be able to find the exact opposite with the same level of authority and expertise. As Dr Douglass declared, "There is no such thing as an undeniable medical fact."

What does this mean for us, those making choices about our health and fitness? Only this—trust yourself and learn to listen to your body. If doing something feels bad, then it most likely is. The endorphins and adrenaline running through the veins of the gym fanatics give them a euphoric kick. Some even develop an addiction to their excessive exercise routine.

Speaking of fitness routines, one condition stands out for me— you must enjoy doing it and get results. If you love going to the gym and working out, that is your choice. If you hate going to gym, if you're looking for an excuse not to go, if you are tired and miserable afterwards, that means you are making the wrong choice.

There are many wonderful physical activities like gardening, dancing, swimming or playing outdoor games. Find what you like and reap a double benefit—your body and soul will enjoy the positive effects of your chosen activity. Recently, a famous German physician, Peter Akst, made a sensational statement: "Fitness and professional sports shorten life." This coincides in a way with a remark by the famously witty Sir Winston Churchill, who apparently said, "I owe my longevity to sport—I've never done any."

Akst, at 76 years of age, is a professor at the University of Applied Sciences in Germany, a doctor of medicine and the author of publications on psychology and gerontology. In his younger years, he used to run long distance. Dr Akst referred to another German professional, a physiologist called Dr Rubner, who established that, at birth, every living being is provided with a certain stock of vital forces which must last their entire lifetime.

Together with his daughter, also a medical doctor, Dr Akst published a book under the provocative title *Lazy Live Longer.* In it, the two doctors referred to the striking and rather shocking examples from the animal kingdom. The average lifespan for the lion, the king of the jungle, whose body is a collection of pumped muscles and who is a fantastic runner, is 8-10 years in a wild savannah, but in a zoo, they live up to 20 years. The polar bear lives in their native Arctic no more than 20 years—in a zoo, their lifetime doubles.

Dr Akst asserted that the major difference is in the animals' lifestyles. In the wild, the animals cover many kilometres a day in search of food, often under stress. On the contrary, in a zoo, animals live in a more relaxed fashion and don't have to fight for survival. They don't use as much energy, nor do they have enemies or competitors, so their life isn't so stressful. Hence, they live twice as long, concluded the professor.

The book further referred to the life of many great athletes who died comparatively young and too often from a heart attack. A sad example was American sports journalist James Fix, the 'god of the marathon and health run'. As the author of the best-selling book *All About Running,* Fix inspired millions around the world to start running. However, he died suddenly during a health run at the age of 52. Even as I was working on this chapter, another sad news story appeared on my TV screen. The Ironman champion and great athlete Dean Mercer died from cardiac arrest while driving. He was 47. That same week, I read an article in the newspaper's Health segment dedicated to untimely heart attacks. One story with the punchline *"My crime? Too much exercise!"* was about Adrian Purtell, 30, a professional rugby player from Leeds, who had a heart attack a few years ago.

"I was the last person you'd expect to have a heart attack. I've been a rugby player since I was 18 and all my life I was committed to staying in shape with rigorous training sessions twice a week." One day, Adrian grossly overexerted himself and was dehydrated—and then it happened. Fortunately, he was quickly transported to the hospital, where, in his words: "after the ECG, I first heard the words 'heart attack'. I was absolutely astonished." It took a year to recover to a point where Adrian could play his favourite sport again, albeit on a smaller scale and now living on a regimen of drugs. In fitness, as in anything else, there are different trends, ideas, beliefs and fads coming and going in and out of practice.

I am not here to take sides. Like in any discussion, there are valid points on either side, for sure. Therefore, I prefer to speak from my own experience. Never forget that you have your own intuition and common sense that can guide you when you are making decisions. That is what I do. During the eight years I worked as a consultant and exercise therapist in my own studio—where my clients were predominantly women over 50—and being a human biologist myself, I came to realise that overexertion is indeed harmful to the body.

My personal story of recovery after a car accident, which caused injuries to my spine and hips, combined with my expertise in human movement, led me to develop my own program. However, the last thing I would do is offer recommendations in this book. Nobody should prescribe medicine or anything else that could affect anyone's health on the pages of any book. That would be totally irresponsible and potentially detrimental to an individual's health, rather than being useful. Therefore, I can only share my personal experience and ideas that cannot and should not be taken as a recommendation without consulting your doctor.

My Routine

A few times a week, I take a 30-minute walk in the fresh air, which is good for both my fitness and my mood. I check my pulse during this time and watch that it stays between 90 and 120 beats per minute. The indication that I'm walking at the right pace is the ability to talk. Not chatting excitedly and loudly, of course, just being able to keep up with a conversation. As soon as my breath becomes intermittent, that's a signal to slow down. So, I allow no puffing, huffing or excessive sweating; just a rhythmic, free movement with swinging arms and pauses, where I will do a few exercises. Younger people could do more, guided by the feeling of a pleasant workout without too much stress on the body.

Stretching is one of the best movements to do on awakening in the morning. I also try to remember to interrupt my sedentary work, whenever my body asks for a good stretch. Two to three times a week I go to a nearby studio equipped with Shapemaster toning beds. This British system suits me brilliantly. It literally brought me back to normal life after my car accident in 2002. I was so impressed and marvelled at my own progress that, when I had a chance, I opened my own studio in Canberra. The power-supported toning beds, developed by a team of sports doctors, engineers, physicians and Pilates practitioners, provides safe and gentle low-to-medium exercise for people of various fitness levels.

> **"To see the brain as a computer helps us to understand how it works and to compare our body with a car teaches us how to look after ourselves."**

It was such an immense pleasure to observe my clients' improvement, sometimes beyond belief. There is no greater satisfaction than seeing their enjoyment and successful results. After selling my studio to a doctor, I myself became a client of a similar studio. In my view, no other system is better suited for mature people. Although the Shapemaster brand has been a leader in the industry for decades, there are now other brands working on the same principles, such as Hypoxy, Slender Me and Hur from Finland. Based on all my countless years of studies and ample scope of expertise, I cannot emphasise strongly enough the importance of not overexerting yourself. Who else will treat you gently and kindly if not you? A bit of laziness from time to time spoiling yourself never hurts.

Therefore, the key word is *balance*—that is, the balance between necessary movement and relaxation. Balance is the universal key to everything in life. Depending on your individual health, lifestyle and circumstances, I hope you find that balance and make any physical activities you partake in a pleasure, not a chore. Pruning your roses, tending to your veggie patch, playing outdoors with your kids or going dancing could not only be beneficial for your body but also a wonderful, joyous, stress-reducing experience.

I'm not trying to discredit formal fitness sessions, say in a swimming pool or gym, don't get me wrong. As I've mentioned before, the fact is that we have made fantastic technological advances and can now see our technical creations as models of ourselves. To see the brain as a computer helps us to understand how it works and to compare our body with a car teaches us how to look after ourselves.

If we use good petrol and oil, take it for regular check-ups, don't rev it up all the time or hit the pedals too hard, our car will serve us for a long time. Imagine doing the opposite, plus putting sugar in the petrol tank—catastrophic! You could always buy another car. It's just a matter of money. However, you cannot buy another body if you treat it carelessly. There is no amount of money in the world that can provide you with a spare body. At least not in this lifetime. It's the only life you've got, it's not a rehearsal. Act accordingly.

How to Make Sensible Choices About Nutrition

Let me start with a statement of ultimate truth beyond any doubt—nutrition is a cornerstone of your health. Nutrition supports all the body's functions and can even be a powerful healing tool. You are what you eat. But as always, the devil is in the detail. If we are lucky, we grow up on proper food and our body goes through the process of growing, getting enough high-quality building materials to lay a foundation for healthy development.

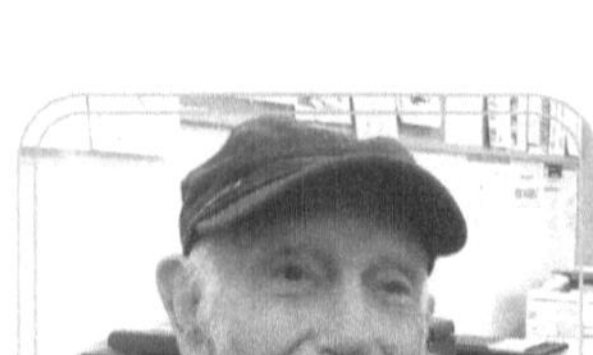When I asked one of my students, Jo Bradley, 96 years old, what he believed to be the reason behind his own longevity, his immediate answer was, "Good parents providing good nutrition." This man is a wonderful example of a clever, humorous and highly capable individual. He continued to say that if you do silly things later in life, like smoking and drinking, not sleeping enough or eating large amounts of junk food, then having a good foundation could get you through those hazards without being as badly affected.

This chapter is not about giving you a list of good products. If I started that conversation, I would never finish. We are all in the same boat trying to avoid foods that are artificial or full of chemicals. We have learned to decipher food labels. Some go organic, although it's expensive and no guarantee of how clean those products really are. I am still wondering how much truth is in those claims, and I have no answer for that. Each of us, therefore, is trying to do their best, especially for our children.

Recently, I visited Cyprus and as I walked into a veggie store, my face was hit by the fantastic smell of the fresh soil, of natural, amazing agricultural produce and a mixture of a huge variety of herbs and spices. I did not know such luxuries still existed. It was a great experience but, unfortunately, it's a rare one. Eating "wrong" brings obesity up. So many people are constantly looking for ways to lose excess weight, which gives so-called "diet gurus" a fantastic source of income. However, we don't need to confuse those "miracle diets" with proper recommendations from professional dieticians.

Dieting is a Trigger for Appetite!

So, let's have a closer look at magic diet pills and other "miracles". My discussion today is about "toxic diets". Why is it that so many diets are often ineffective? You can lose the weight but find it difficult to keep it off. Some of them can even

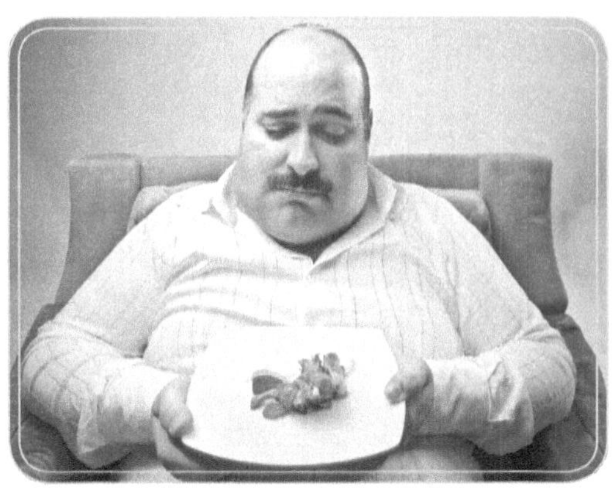

damage your health irreparably. If these diets are supposed to work wonders, then why is the population getting fatter?

Let's look at the pros and cons. Why is it so difficult to sustain weight loss after going off the diet? Any diet is both physiologically and mentally stressful. Therefore, your body will attempt to compensate for the loss, so it can get back to its initial state. Then it stores a bit more fat just in case the owner of this body decides again to force it to starve.

On a diet, our body loses a long list of biologically valuable components—fats, complex carbs, etc.—that we consider to be bad for us. If you continue consuming only, say, 1,200 calories a day, then gradually your metabolism begins to play up, hypovitaminosis kicks in and all body systems suffer. Interestingly, our mind reacts to any prohibition by increasing desire. The necessity to control yourself makes you irritable and unhappy. A person on a diet lives in a permanent state of stress, producing excessive amounts of the hormone cortisol.

The shorter and stricter your diet, the higher the risk of piling it all back on. Research proves that, after a one-week strict diet, the risk is 95%, while after a longer dieting regime, it would be no more than 10%. Based on scientific evidence, these are the worst kinds of diets.

1.   PROTEIN DIETS

These are based on the expectation that, after a while, the human body—which is not designed to function properly without carbs—will start using its own fatty deposits as a substitute for carbs and that is how you start losing weight. However, it is extremely harmful for your metabolism. This is an unbearable load for your kidneys that suffer tremendously as they work to excrete the colossal amount of protein. Plus, attempting to process such large amounts of protein is tough on the digestion, especially in the absence of fibre. Your mouth smells of ammonia and your sweat stinks. You feel tired, lethargic and nauseous. That is too high a price for losing weight, which will inevitably come back.

2.   LOW-FAT DIETS

These diets are based on the exclusion of fats, including the good fats found in fish, olives and avocado. These are what protect us from atherosclerosis. They are necessary for the brain and the general balance of our system. Lack of fat is reflected in the condition of our hair and nails. Plus, without fats, vitamins A, D, E and K are not properly absorbed and digested.

3.   ONE-PRODUCT DIETS (MONO DIETS)

From time to time, these come into fashion. A popular one is the rice diet, when you eat only rice, no salt or any seasoning. Eat as much as you wish, and drink only water. Other varieties used are cottage cheese, apples or grapefruit—the list goes on. On these diets, fat deposits literally melt in front of your eyes. The body becomes catastrophically undernourished of important substances. As a result, conditions like anaemia and osteopenia—the loss of bone minerals—develop rapidly. The immune system suffers, and your body's defences fail.

4.   EXPRESS DIETS

These allow you to lose up to five kilograms in three to five days. You essentially starve yourself. Breakfast is a piece of cheese and a coffee, no sugar. Lunch is 100 grams of meat and some veggies, and dinner is just a mint tea. By the end of the first day, you get a headache, you have no energy and you're in a bad mood. However, in a few days, your favourite dress fits you again. Then the effect is gone, and you are back to square one.

5.   CLEANSING DIETS

These diets consist of either raw vegetables or cereal soaked in water. This one is supposed to work as a sponge, cleansing our intestines from some mysterious toxic deposits. The recommended duration for this diet is 10-14 days and you are supposed to feel like a new-born baby. Unfortunately, that is not really what happens. Firstly, the coarse food is bad for many people, leading to flatulence and diarrhoea. The cereals being already digested in the stomach cannot "cleanse" anything in the colon.

I could carry on but, in a nutshell, you need to make the right choice, preferably under your doctor's supervision. Some diets are rational and can be helpful, especially as a kick-start to weight loss. Others are just absurd. As I once read, "Monday: a spoon of rice, Wednesday: a cabbage leaf, Saturday: cremation." Now, enough negativity. Let's find out how we can get a slender figure the right way.

According to specialists such as dieticians, endocrinologists, gastroenterologists and physicians, we shouldn't starve or deprive ourselves. Rather, we should implement lifestyle changes, especially in our eating habits. Our common, modern diets are increasingly low in four important nutrients that have a direct bearing on ageing, which has a negative effect on the brain. If you hope to one day be a healthy and happy centenarian, the most important supplements are vitamin D, DHA, folic acid and magnesium.

The famous Japanese doctor, Shigeaki Hinohara, who lived and worked to the age of 105, left behind his 11-point recommendation on how to live a happy and healthy life. The number one item on his list says, "Eat less."

So, instead of fancy diets, we need to eat quality food in smaller portions. No miracle solutions, no magic pills. It is the only fair deal on offer. But, for the first step, we need to change our mindset. Logically, if we accumulate excessive weight through decades or at least years, how can we realistically expect to get rid of it with the wave of a hand?

"As soon as we decide how to change our eating habits, we are on the road to success."

The good thing is that, with time and effort, we can lose excessive weight gently and gradually, and most importantly, stay healthy and in good shape. As soon as we decide how to change our eating habits, we are on the road to success—and long-term success, not the delusional flash of fantasy. Slow and steady enjoys the best results.

When speaking about nutrition with people who wish to live a long and happy life, the inevitable weight loss conversation comes up. This global problem is frightening, with a rapidly growing number of overweight people. My family, friends and clients often discuss it, sometimes arguing which diet is better or how much exercise is needed to keep excessive weight at bay. We all know that to make steps and achieve results, one needs motivation. I wish to share an example from my practice.

Marta, a client of mine in her early fifties, was grossly overweight, to such a degree that if she did not start doing something immediately, her health would have been under serious threat. She realised this and was looking for help. She said her motivation was strong and she just needed some help and support but when I started asking questions, it became very clear that her motivation was in fact quite weak. I had to explain to her that she needed to clearly understand what she wanted to change, in precise terms, and what she would be striving to achieve. She had a general picture but when it came to the details, it took some time to get to the core of the problem. Our chat went something like this:

"Marta," I said, "do you know why you want to lose weight?"

"What a strange question!" she replied. "Of course, I know—my weight is my problem!"

"And how is it a problem? How does it affect you?"

"Well," she continued, "I look ugly, I don't get to wear nice clothing. People judge me and make nasty comments."

"Okay," I replied. "Is that all? If they stopped making comments and you could fit into a lovely dress, would all your problems be solved?"

She paused for a moment.

"No, of course not."

"Then what else? How is your obesity the problem?"

"Well, I can't walk without puffing," she replied, "and I have to stop after a few steps. I can't breathe properly even with slight movements."

Now we were getting down to it.

"So, the problem is in your breathing?" I carried on. "You just want to breathe easier, right?"

"No, not just that! I take lots of medication—for blood pressure, cholesterol, my heart…"

"So, you want to lose weight so that you can breathe better, stop taking your medication and not get nasty comments—is that all?"

"Oh, no, it's much bigger … let me think."

This was good—she wanted to think, and she needed to think hard. It was just what I wanted to hear because just starting up a diet and getting results is quite possible, but it simply isn't enough. Without processing it in her own mind or changing her mindset towards a healthy life for the rest of her days, her weight would come back with a vengeance. Only the understanding of what her goal is would help her win the battle in the long term.

Before people realise what the negative consequences of obesity are, and what positive benefits they gain by losing excessive weight, they only have a vague idea which cannot support strong motivation. So, to move from a general understanding to a strong motivation, I ask my clients to list ten negative consequences of being overweight in relation to their health, relationships, social environment, work, prosperity, personal development, the joy of life and spirituality. Then, I ask them to list ten positive consequences of losing weight.

Therefore, when answering both groups of questions, a person begins to see a complete picture of how carrying so much weight is negatively impacting their life and the positivity they would achieve with a slimmer and healthier lifestyle. That is their moment of truth—the moment a new program is being created in their subconscious.

Night Food

As we intend to eat less, we can do so by having smaller portions and not eating after 6 pm. Another way to reduce our appetite is to inhale nice but neutral aromas like vanilla, green apple or cinnamon. Such aromas suppress our appetite as they directly impact our brain's emotional sectors. We can usually handle our appetite well until the evening.

Then, somehow, we feel an urge to check our fridge. It often starts with an innocent cup of tea but ends up with an accompanying sandwich, a couple of cookies or a lovely piece of cake. Of course, it feels great. However, we pay for those pleasurable moments later.

Unfortunately, consuming those small delights, we're only topping up our fat deposits. To fight human nature's call for night food is a difficult task. Recently, dieticians released some recommendations for those who cannot resist that call and suggested what foods are suitable for late snacking. These choices improve the quality of your sleep and don't move the arrow on your scales further to the right. Here they are—five safe night snacks.

DARK CHOCOLATE: It contains a minimal amount of sugar and helps to reduce your cholesterol level. A couple of squares would be okay.

SOUP: Any warm liquids are relaxing and calming. It could be chicken or vegetable—however, lentil or pea soups are not recommended as they can lead to disturbed sleep.

ALMONDS: A handful of almonds can satisfy your appetite while not causing weight gain.

PUMPKIN SEEDS: If your hand is reaching out for a packet of popcorn or chips, try pumpkin seeds instead. They are rich in magnesium, which supports a quiet, deep sleep.

RICE: Dieticians believe that diets based on rice diminish the risk of insomnia by 46%. Rice has a high GI that encourages the production of tryptophan and melatonin. These hormones are highly beneficial for a good night's sleep.

Also, we must understand our body's tricks. Often, when we feel hungry we are in fact thirsty. So, before grabbing a snack, have a glass of water or a nice, warm ginger tea.

Water—The Greatest Healer of All

Water is our life force. With a glass in hand, let's refresh what we know about this miracle drink. Water is energy, the best electrolyte ever. A glass of fresh, pure water beats any commercial electrolyte drink. Without water, our cellular powerhouse—also known as mitochondria—can't supply our cells with energy. The first organ that suffers because of a lack of water is our brain. Not drinking enough shows through irritability, headaches, migraines, fatigue and a lack of concentration.

> **"Water is energy, the best electrolyte ever. A glass of fresh, pure water beats any commercial electrolyte drink."**

We know our daily amount of water intake should be between one-and-a-half and three litres. The amount widely depends on your age, condition, physical activities, etc. However, not everybody knows how to take it. For the best benefit, we need to drink water on an empty stomach, at least 10-15 minutes before a meal. This allows it to easily pass through the stomach and reach the area near the duodenum, where the water becomes alkalised. Being alkaline is very beneficial to the body.

Instead of paying money for bottled water, we can prepare perfect, pure water at home for free. We just need to collect tap water in a three-litre jar and leave it overnight. The next day, carefully pour out about two-thirds into a pan, leaving a residue at the bottom of the jar. Put the pan with the tap water on a hot stove and wait until the first small bubbles appear. Switch it off. This is called "cold boiling water". Doing so preserves its structure for 24 hours. I would put the purity of your drinking water as priority number one. You can also buy good quality water from stores—just check what's in it carefully.

Water can also be an external healer, cleaning, refreshing and moisturising the body. Using contrast temperature water can stop an asthma attack and relieve a high blood pressure crisis. In both cases, you need two bowls—one with hot, but tolerable, water and the other one with cold water. Put your hands in the hot bowl for ten seconds, then swiftly place them into the cold for another ten seconds. Keep alternating your hands up to twenty times, ending up in the hot one. The change of temperature makes your blood vessels contract and release, which is beneficial for the bronchial system's asthmatic spasms and for blood circulation. Ideally the same can be done with your feet. Hot and cold water has many uses.

As a curious example of an extreme use of cold water, for the whole nineteenth century in Germany, ice water was a popular treatment for rheumatism. Sometimes patients even had to break a layer of ice in to submerge themselves in the water, it was that cold. The most amazing thing was that the treatment worked. In Northern Europe and North America, cold water treatments are still popular. In Russia, especially in Siberia, kids run naked and roll in the snow. After getting hot in a sauna, people jump into icy water. These people are rarely subjected to colds and flu. They usually do it in large groups and then appropriately polish off their cold dip with a hot tea and a shot of vodka.

Nine Signs You're Not Drinking Enough Water

There is no need to talk about the importance of water for the body, which is made up of 70% water. However, if we forget to get enough water during the day, we deprive our body of that vital resource. No other liquid is a replacement for pure water. All liquids contain water but to separate it and make it usable for your metabolism is a job for your cells that required the expenditure of energy. So, if you notice one of the signs I have listed below, please replenish yourself as soon as possible.

Dryness In The Mouth And Skin

When we feel that dryness, we know we need to have a drink of water. However, sweet or fizzy drinks do not solve our hydration problems—only water can do that. Dry skin is the earliest sign of dehydration, which can lead to serious consequences. Lack of water in the skin means a lack of sweating. In turn, the body is losing its ability to excrete dirt and some fat that needs to be removed daily. The solution, of course, is to drink more pure water.

Extreme Thirst After Drinking Alcohol

This is not the same as dryness in the mouth. Anyone who has ever experience a hangover knows how bad it feels when after awakening you cannot quench your thirst. Alcohol can totally dehydrate you, so your body and mind transmit an urgent SOS—don't ignore it!

Dry Eyes

Dry eyes are a sign that there is a lack of water in your tear ducts. It is damaging to your eyes, especially for those who use contact lenses.

Painful Joints

Did you know that joint pain could be exacerbated, or even caused by dehydration? Our joints and cartilage need moisture for protection, to avoid them grinding against each other at every step. That is why it is so important to keep joints hydrated by drinking plenty of water, especially if you suffer from conditions like arthritis, gout or a joint injury. With a proper water balance in the body, our joints can absorb the shock from sharp movements like running, jumping or awkward falls.

Sickness Lasts Longer

Our organs work hard to filter out toxins. However, this mechanism cannot function properly without water. When dehydrated, our organs begin sucking water from our blood and lymphatic system, which makes you feel sicker for longer.

Tiredness And Lethargy

When the body begins to "borrow" water from our blood, we receive a reduced oxygen supply to our organs. This manifests as tiredness and drowsiness that even coffee can't fix.

Extreme Hunger

The signals for dehydration feel the same as the signals for hunger. Therefore, if you feel hungry, have a drink of water first and then decide whether you really need to eat. For some people, this happens a lot at night. So, instead of going right to the kitchen and opening the fridge, try some water.

Digestion Problems

As well as feeling dryness in our mouth, a similar dryness in the stomach leads to a diminishing amount and thickness of mucus. In turn, gastric acid erodes the internal walls of our stomach and intestines. This is one of the common causes of reflux and an upset stomach.

Early Signs Of Ageing

The amount of water our body can hold gets smaller with age. That is why we need to increase our water consumption as we age. It's very important to set up a routine and not just rely on memory. For example, a two-litre jug filled with water every morning will help to keep you hydrated. We know we've done well when, by the evening, the jug is empty.

It's better to have more water than less—make it a rule. Why not has a glass right now?

A Myth About Salt

If you're in your seventies or beyond, there is a chance that your doctor has attributed your feeling of fatigue, your balance problems or sometimes dizziness to the fact that you are "getting older". However, the real culprit could be a low level of sodium in the blood, called hyponatraemia. Several years ago, research showed that a surprising number of seniors suffer from this. It occurs because many elderly people have avoided salt throughout their lives, having been told it was a cause of high blood pressure. However, on the contrary, low sodium intake may actually increase a risk of heart attack and death.

In my practice, working with seniors, I have constantly warned them against not having enough salt in their diet. However, they were understandably sceptical. I tried to persuade them to start using salt in small amounts with little success. One day, Bronwyn, one of my clients who had not been well for a while, went for a medical check-up where she received a hyponatrae-mia diagnosis. For so many years she had avoided salt like the plague, thinking she was doing the right thing—and now she was paying the price.

In his reports on this subject, Dr McCarron, a professor at the University of California stated, "There's currently no reliable evidence that supports the recommendation to reduce intake of salt for heart health. My view is that it is very likely that low salt will ultimately prove to be another public health disaster. There is already sufficient evidence to suggest that low salt could actually result in an increased risk of cardiovascular disease."

Sleepless at Night

"Good Sleep, Healthy Ageing" — this is a slogan used when the world celebrates World Sleep Day, a global event that occurs annually on the second Friday of March. It is organised by the World Sleep Society, formerly the World Association of Sleep Medicine. So, why is regular daily sleep so important? A few days without sleep can irreparably affect the human body. People start hallucinating, they lose consciousness and—if sleeplessness continues—they can even die. But why is this? Let's compare sleep with other vital necessities.

Without air, we can live for only a few minutes, best-case scenario. The current world record for holding breath in water without moving is 11 minutes and 35 seconds and was set by Stéphane Mifsud in 2009. However, for an average person, it is no more than five minutes before convulsions and loss of consciousness begin. This happens because when the brain experiences a lack of oxygen, all body functions cease, leading to death.

So, what about water? How long can we go without this vital fluid that comprises two-thirds of our bodies? Without water, we can survive just a few days. In a comfortable environment, however, an adult can last without water for around a week.

Without food, which is a source of energy, a person could live much longer, maybe a few weeks, using the body's own deposits. An Irish political prisoner, Terence MacSwiney, whose 74-day strike ended with his death in 1920, undertook the longest-lasting hunger strike in recorded history. All three deprivations can be explained logically. Air, water and food are necessary for our survival and for sustaining our body's functions.

But what about sleep?

When one goes without sleep for 20 to 25 hours, their behaviour becomes like that of someone with a blood-alcohol level of 0.1 percent. Up to 72 hours without sleep, your body and mind operate in altered states, mixing up reality with illusion. Then, physiological changes develop in the brain. That's when your health and your life are in mortal danger. A good night's sleep is one of life's blessings. As Coleridge wrote years ago, "Oh, sleep! It is a gentle thing, beloved from pole to pole." Wilse Webb, a prominent sleep researcher, more recently called sleep 'the gentle tyrant' — it can be delayed but not defeated. We spend about 25 years of our lives in a sleeping state, with a quarter of this time spent dreaming.

A healthy person's sleep pattern is based on a 24-hour cycle. How long we sleep depends on our age. Kids need 10-11 hours of sleep daily, adolescents 9-10, adults 7-8 and, in older people, 6-7 hours can be enough. The best time for sleeping is proven to be before midnight, around 10-11pm. We all have dreams while sleeping but if we do not write them down as soon as we wake up, 90% will be forgotten within half an hour.

Chronic lack of sleep—less than six hours a night—can affect your vision and hearing and increase anxiety. Physiological conditions such as nervous ticks, loss of concentration, apathy and general weakness, metabolic deviations and rapid weight gain can also develop. Not sleeping at all for a few days will cause visual and auditory hallucinations, loss of objective reality, then paranoid behaviour and eventually death.

> **"A good night's sleep is one of life's blessings."**

Why do we suffer so badly? It is not just about tiredness or a lack of rest. There is something else which, is still not fully understood. Sleep is a mysterious state of the body and mind. Many stories, myths and unexplainable facts regarding sleep have remained unsolved for centuries.

In many parts of the world, people believe that dreams can be prophetic. In some traditional societies in Africa, dreams are considered so important that people make decisions about marriages, justice and even war based on their dreams. Many scientific discoveries have been made in the sleeping state. This is explained by the fact that, during sleep, our brain interprets information that is already there in a completely different way. Take nuclear physicist Niels Bohr, who discovered the structure of the atom in his dream, as well as the chemist Friedrich Kekule, who discovered the formula for benzene.

The Russian chemical scientist Dmitry Mendeleev made the most striking scientific discovery, the periodic table, in his sleep. Another example was Richard Wagner, a composer, who insisted that his famous opera, *Tristan and Isolde*, was given to him during his sleep. Current theory says that, during the day, various malfunctions occur in the body. If they are not fixed in good time, the consequences can be catastrophic. The mighty unconscious has enormous capabilities that our imagination cannot even grasp but, at the same time, it is subservient to our conscious mind. Once a day, the unconscious mind sends its host to sleep to have quiet, uninterrupted time to diagnose and repair any damage.

It has been shown that, during sleep, our metabolism works on creating new cells and tissues. Our whole body is being rejuvenated. If it is deprived of this and cannot perform this work, that's where the trouble starts. In some cultures, mainly situated in warmer climates, a daytime sleep, or "siesta", is very popular. It was discovered that regular, daytime sleep could decrease the risk of cardiovascular diseases. Our body appreciates even small portions of sleep. For example, according to Dr Douglass, "Napping is fabulous medicine." Winston Churchill, Thomas Edison, Napoleon, JFK and other human dynamos shared this sleepy little secret that can make you smarter, sexier and more productive.

While napping is a nice, relaxing thing to do, another kind of short sleep is dangerous. I am talking about "micro-sleep". It lasts for a few seconds and always comes suddenly. It is caused by a lack of night sleep, fatigue or depression. The danger is that it can happen while you are driving or working with complex, technical equipment. In relation to longevity, it would be of great benefit to us to set up some napping time during our day if we could. Providing so many benefits including refreshing our vision, supporting our heart, giving us energy and relaxing our nerves, who wouldn't want an afternoon siesta?

Second Morning

I'm sure I don't need to convince you that our wellbeing depends on our energy levels. We have known this for ages and of course, we notice that, at certain times of the day, our energy levels drop significantly. I'm sure you have experienced it yourself. We are talking about the after-lunch slump. Our personal productivity depends on two major factors:

- The quality of our sleep.

- Topping up our energy during the day.

The afternoon slump happens because our body is gradually losing its charge. Unfortunately, we usually use stimulants like coffee or a sugar hit. However, it doesn't last long—after all, these are not natural sources of energy and often require repeated doses. Mother Nature, caring as always, has a much better option. Exactly seven hours after waking up, we need to perform a reloading of our bio-system. That number did not fall from the sky but rather is a result of serious scientific exploration. It has been proven that a decline in energy levels begins at that exact time after we wake up—seven hours.

Therefore, that is the point where we need to recharge our batteries. It is well known that a huge portion of our daily energy, approximately 70 percent, is spent using our eyes. Consequently, seven hours after waking, we start losing the energy we have built up overnight. The solution? We need to shut our eyes for about 20 minutes. I know it sounds simple, but this is the best energy uploading process—it really works! When we close our eyes and give them a 20-minute rest, our body automatically switches from one regime to another, meaning it stops spending energy and begins accumulating it.

One obvious issue with this process is the risk of falling asleep. That's not good. Firstly, you cannot fall asleep at work. Secondly, a long nap could defeat the purpose—it does not lift your energy but rather relaxes you even more. Also, the quality of your sleep could suffer later as well. The best way to avoid this is to listen to some motivating or energetic music. The benefit of this method is that, when we open our eyes, it is like experiencing a second morning in the afternoon, where we are full of energy again, ready to be productive and cheerful, whether we're at work or at home.

Try it for yourself!

Memory and Mnemonic Training

*"We are what we repeatedly do.
Excellence, then, is not an act, but a habit."*

— Aristotle

As I mentioned earlier, mnemonics is techniques for memory training. Let's look at some of the tools that we have at our disposal. There are plenty of recommendations, suggestions and mental exercises. One simple way is to make a routine of daily revision.

Basic memory training can be easily performed without preparation. According to Dr Tatiana Chernigovskaya, a Russian scientist in the field of neuroscience, psycholinguistics and the theory of the mind, "Memory training should be child's play, not a torture."

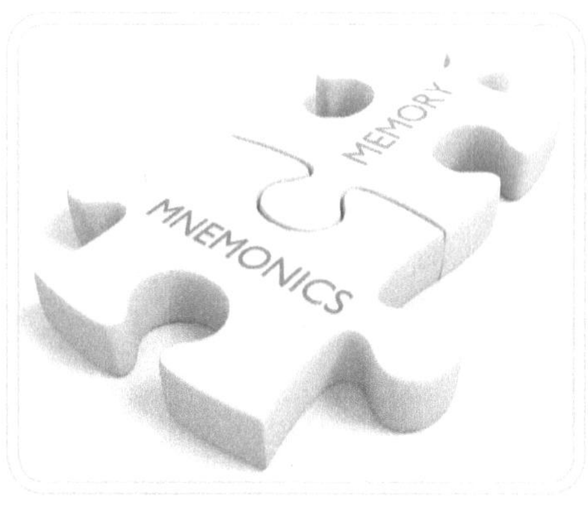

Here are a few exercises to strengthen your memory. Remember though, don't push it too hard. The more often you make your mental mechanisms register and reproduce things that you wish to memorise, the easier it becomes. Repetition is the key to any training.

Exercise 1

This is an excellent exercise for training your memory, attention, awareness and mindfulness, and it puts your neurological connections in order. At night, before falling asleep, try remembering everything that happened to you since the moment you woke up. You may close your eyes for better concentration.

Slowly, recall all the details of your day—getting up, putting your slippers on, going to the bathroom, brushing your teeth, etc. Visualise the colour of your toothbrush and towel.

Then, what did you wear, how was your breakfast, where did you go and what did you do throughout the day? Who did you talk to? Did you call someone, did someone call you? Process all the day's events in as much detail as you can.

Exercise 2

Take a list of 16 words. For instance, "chair, table, soup, letter, car, ocean, apple, beacon, cork, tram, shoes, wardrobe, house, boat, camping and piano". Read and explore these words for 90 seconds. Then write down as many as you can remember.

If you can remember less than nine that means that you don't use your memory enough. Repeat the process in an hour, don't re-check the list and see how many you get. You might surprise yourself and get a better result. Try associating the words with images in your mind.

Exercise 3

Before you go to sleep, make yourself a memory training plan for tomorrow. For example, look at the vase that is standing on the glass console table by the window. Take a mental picture of it. Decide that tomorrow at 7 pm you will move this vase to the top of your bookcase. Don't write it down anywhere. Don't ask anybody to remind you.

The next day, at 7 pm sharp, take the vase and put it on the bookcase. Believe it or not, this is a difficult task. If you do it on the first attempt, that's great. If you forget, don't beat yourself up—set it up again and see how it works out the second time. Keep going until you get it.

Exercise 4

Another excellent way to improve your nervous system's workings, including memorising, is to listen to classical music, sounds of nature or jazz. Researchers consider listening to music as one of the most important tools for relaxing the mind and improving the memory. Music, at its essence, is what triggers memories.

Your ability to concentrate and stay focused underpins the workings of your memory. This is of paramount importance. Concentration leads to memorising and requires full attention on the subject, allowing no other thoughts to interfere. Below are two training techniques for improving concentration.

Exercise 5

Take an object like a watch, a pen or a bunch of keys. Observe it carefully for 30 seconds, then close your eyes and try to see it with your inner vision in every detail. Start with simple objects and then choose more complex ones as your concentration improves.

Exercise 6

Switch on your TV or radio—the news is quite good for this—and gradually decrease the volume, until you are just able to understand the speech. The low-intensity sound will increase your level of concentration on the sound. Do this for up to three minutes at a time.

Exercise 7

Mnemonics is an exercise where you train both your brain and memory. You can do it with friends and family, make it challenging, funny or even ridiculous, which sometimes makes it even easier to memorise. Let's look at some examples that you might already know:

How to memorise the order of planets: My Very Excited Mother Just Served Us Ninety Pies. Mercury, Venus, Earth, Mars, Jupiter, Saturn, Uranus, Neptune and Pluto.

How to memorise the year when Columbus sailed to America: Columbus sailed the ocean blue, in fourteen hundred ninety-two.

It's great fun to create your own mnemonics and improve your memorising skills at the same time.

Natural Remedies

This section was the most challenging for me. I have in my possession so many recipes, ideas, stories and recommendations that to choose favourites has been extremely tough. In my field of expertise, I consider home remedies to be not only things like herbs, essences, natural therapies or folk medicine but also

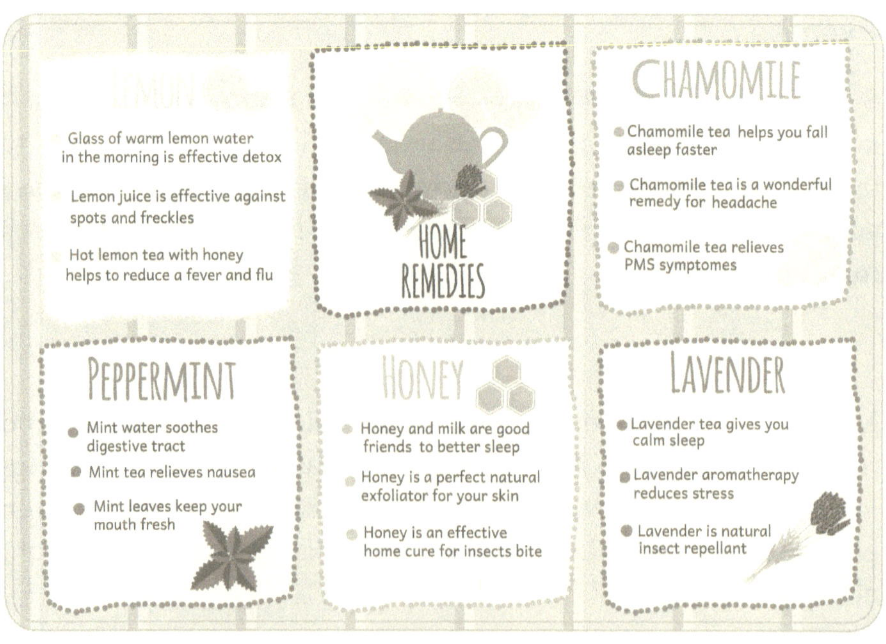

activities you can do to improve your health. I have based my choices on simplicity, affordability and availability.

I cannot emphasise strongly enough that nobody can treat, heal or cure a person just by giving general advice or their opinion. Therefore, what you read in this book is just food for thought. I'd like to start off with some home remedies that you can use that may already be sitting in your pantry or medicine cabinet. They are bicarbonate of soda, salt and iodine.

Mother Nature has been generous to us since the beginning of time, providing many natural means for treating an array of health conditions. But the more expensive and often harmful chemicals we pop in our medicine cabinets, the less we rely on Mother Nature's gifts. What's remarkable, in a strange way, is that most of us know those natural secrets—but what we know and what we do are two different things. Natural remedies take time to do their job and deliver results. It is much easier to use a quick fix from the medicine cabinet. We're so conditioned to do this that we turn a blind eye to the possibility of harmful side effects. We just want it all and we want it now, no matter the consequences.

Nowadays, it's so easy to Google and discover the power of bicarbonate of soda and the many other wonderful substances with proven healing properties. My message to you is simply that there are many better, healthier and much cheaper ways to treat some conditions than to go straight to powerful but sometimes dangerous man-made chemicals.

Bicarbonate of Soda—A Miracle Mineral

Bicarbonate of soda has been used in both official medicine and home remedies since ancient times. Nowadays, its efficacy for treating many conditions and ailments has been confirmed in a large amount of reputable research.

Its first exceptionally useful property is that it alkalises the body. The alkalising process could be as simple as having a quarter of a teaspoon of soda with warm water before you go to sleep. Half a teaspoon in hot milk with honey soothes a sore throat and reduces a cough while gargling with soda and salt in warm water promotes healing in the throat. You know all this, but the question remains—do we follow what we know, or do we just grab something from the chemist without a second thought?

Bicarbonate of soda can also be used for the treatment of burns by flame, hot surfaces or acid. Simply rinse the affected area with a baking soda solution, then cover it with a cloth soaked in the same solution.

This miracle mineral can be used topically to treat haemorrhoids, Whitlow (an inflammation of the fingers), conjunctivitis, fungal infections and eczema. It can be consumed in water to treat arrhythmia attacks or acid reflux, gargled to cure a toothache, pharyngitis or laryngitis, or even applied to the underarms to rid them of unpleasant odour-causing bacteria. You can also put a baking soda solution in a steam inhaler and breath in the vapour to treat a cough or other respiratory problems.

More about salt

Apart from being a food product, salt has amazing healing properties. Let's check some of them. Take common salt, as an example. A 1:10 salt-water solution can be used for cleaning wounds and injuries, gargling and clearing the nose, refreshing the internal mucous lining and supporting better breathing. In yoga practices, it is recommended as a preventive and cleansing measure for protecting our respiratory system. As an anti-bacterial agent, salt can be used for treating cuts and wounds by applying a cloth saturated in the solution directly.

During the Second World War, in Russian military hospitals, surgeons used water from the Barents Sea as a natural bactericidal solution. There was a shortage of antibiotics and medications, but the trusty saline solution saved hundreds of soldiers' lives. After a few days under saline bandages, wounds would be cleared of pus and fever would subside.

The fact is that the saline solution absorbs discharge with its pathogenic microbial content, and sucks out all the dirt and toxins, clearing the wounds. With all the arsenal of medications available from the chemist, we tend not to bother with natural solutions. But health-conscious people often ask themselves: what are the actual content

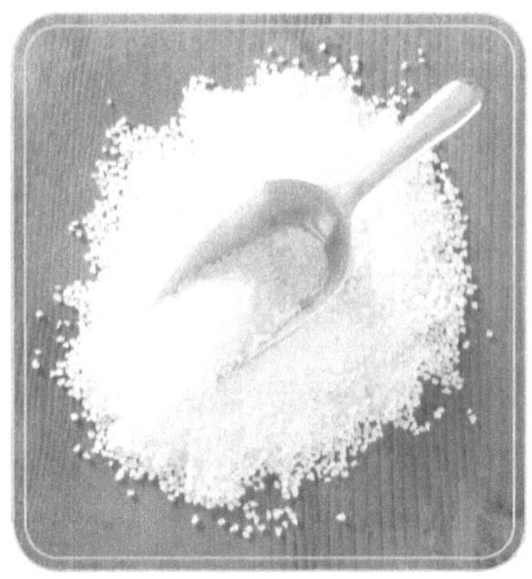

of these medications? Are they based on hormones, antibiotics or strong chemicals? Are they human-friendly substances? How do we know? In my view, it is time to get back to basics.

Mother Nature is kind to us. She has gifts for us, including clever remedies against many ailments. Natural and folk therapy treatments are easily available and simple to use. Saline solution can relieve inflammation, clear our nose and throat, and heal cuts and wounds.

Iodine

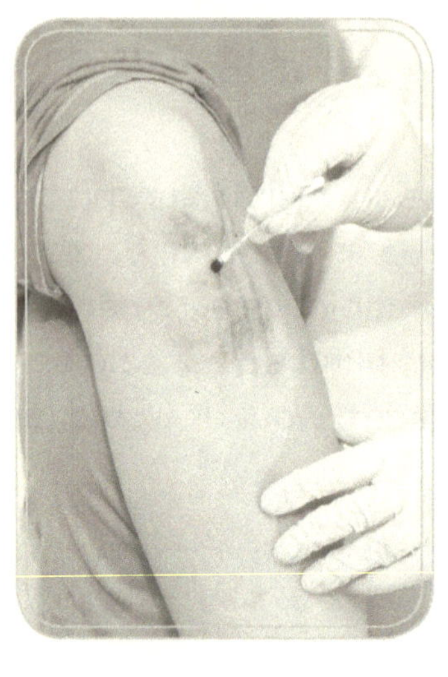

Iodine tincture is also known as Betadine. It's a chemical element that is required for growth and survival. An iodine deficiency can lead to goitre, a disease characterised by an abnormally enlarged thyroid gland, which leads to some serious health consequences. Iodine tincture in alcohol is one of the most effective and easily available antiseptics. However, iodine can also be used for treating a whole range of conditions.

A few inter-crossing lines (the so-called "iodine grid") drawn on the skin helps relieve malaise because of the double effect of iodine on the body. Firstly, iodine molecules strengthen local blood flow, creating a heat-producing effect. Secondly, by entering subcutaneous tissues via the pores, iodine suppresses bacterial activities and reduces the intensity of inflammation.

Other conditions that could benefit from using the iodine grid include:

- Respiratory conditions
- Varicose veins

- Injuries and bruises

- Back and joint pain

- Iodine deficiency

In developed countries, people usually get enough iodine from their food. However, this may not be the case for some people with metabolic disorders or pregnant women.

Salvation for Your Knee Joints

One of the most common complaints is knee pain. They're the most hard-working joints, subjected to a lot of wear and tear through the years. With age, our ligaments and connected tissues gradually lose their elasticity and mobility. This brings discomfort and pain, especially while walking. Due to various factors, especially poor nutrition, the production and viscosity of the synovial liquid in the joints diminishes. This is a direct road to arthroses.

To prevent further inflammation and destruction there are natural recipes to strengthen your knees without medication and surgery. This oat drink is useful for anybody who suffers from knee pain. It strengthens synovial liquid production and improves the elasticity of ligaments in the joints. The ingredients are:

- 1 glass of water

- 50g of oat flakes

- 100ml of orange juice

- 1 tablespoon of crushed nuts

- ➡ 1 tablespoon of honey

- ➡ Cinnamon to taste

Cook the porridge using the oats and water as normal. Once it has cooled, mix in the rest of ingredients and blend. This cocktail is rich in nutrients that support the normalisation of the metabolism and synovial liquid production.

Seven recipes for Brain Vessel Cleansing

As we strive for healthy longevity we need to look after our memory and our mind. Health-wise, that means taking good care of our brain's blood vessels. With time, some unwanted deposits accumulate on the inside walls, blood circulation gradually begins to experience difficulties and the workings of our brain become disrupted.

We can help using herbal remedies that we can make at home. There are a few examples of herbal infusions that demonstrate their efficacy through centuries. These remedies make our vessels soft and non-rigid, eliminate dizziness and noise in the ears, improve metabolism and support general body cleansing.

Herbal Infusion For Brain Vessels Cleansing

- ➡ 100g of camomile

- ➡ 100g of St John's Wort

- ➡ 100g of immortelle

- ➡ 100g of birch buds

- ➡ Water

⮕ Honey

⮕ Bay rum oil

Shred the herbs and mix them up. Boil half a litre of water and pour it over 1 tablespoon of the mixture, leaving it to brew for 20 minutes. Then strain it, take half of the liquid, add 1 teaspoon of honey and 1 drop of bay rum oil. Drink it last thing before going to sleep.

The next morning, warm up the rest of the liquid but do not re-boil. Add another teaspoon of honey and another drop of bay rum oil. Drink it 20 minutes before breakfast. Keep making this concoction and use it as above every day until all herbs are used. Like with any natural medicine, results can take time, but you should feel it after 2-3 weeks.

One more recipe came from a nurse who suggested it to some patients in the haematology ward where she worked. She also recommended it for after chemotherapy to restore the immune system, especially for kids. This mixture covers a much wider range of conditions including kidney and cardiovascular problems, atrophy of the optic nerve, cramps in the legs and more. So strong is the power of pine needles, the main ingredient of the recipe.

Preparation For Brain Vessel Restoration Based On Pine Needles

⮕ 5 tablespoon of pine needles

⮕ 2 tablespoons of crushed rosehip berries

⮕ 2 tablespoons of onion husks

⮕ 1 litre of water

Mix the ingredients together and bring to boil—leave to brew overnight wrapped in a warm blanket. Drink between half a litre and one litre daily.

A Very Simple Remedy

This remedy should be used for a long time, no less than 3 months. Every morning you eat a mandarin, a small handful of raisins and three walnuts, exactly in that order. Don't mix them or chew them together. Then don't consume any other food or drink for 20 minutes. After this time has elapsed, have a glass of water and continue with your proper breakfast. The success of this remedy depends on it being used every day, precisely as described.

Brain Vessel Cleansing With Garlic

- 1 bulb of garlic
- 1 glass of unrefined sunflower oil
- 1 lemon
- 1 teaspoon of garlic oil

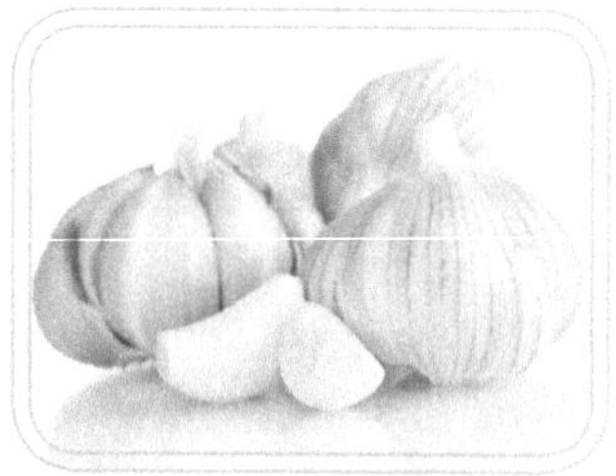

Take the garlic, press it and cover with the sunflower oil, then put it in the fridge. The next day, juice the lemon. Mix the garlic oil with a teaspoon of lemon juice and take it 30 minutes before meals, three times per day. However, don't mix them in advance. The course of this treatment is a minimum of one month.

Lemon, Orange And Honey Remedy

This is a very useful recipe for cleansing the vessels in the brain and strengthening the immune system. Plus, it is beneficial for your nervous system. Take 2 lemons and 2 oranges—remove the pips but keep the skin—mince or blend them into a homogeneous mass. Place into a glass jar, add 2 tablespoons of honey and refrigerate. Take 2 teaspoons of this citrus honey before a meal over the course of a month. It is very tasty and full of goodness.

Ruby Grapefruit Solution

This is a well-known and proven method for cleansing your vessels. Grapefruit has some unique properties that make it the perfect food to enjoy while you're getting rid of the toxins in your body. If you start your breakfast with a half a grapefruit—preferably the ruby variety—for a month, you will feel the difference.

"Elixir Of Life"

This is an easy recipe for cleansing the vessels, eliminating headaches and supporting general wellbeing. Take honey, olive oil and lemon juice in equal proportion (1:1:1). Mix them and take 1 teaspoon of the mixture every morning on an empty stomach, 30 minutes before breakfast—that's it.

Many people, including my friends and relatives, with great success, have used all these recipes. Try them for yourself!

The Easiest Remedy to Rejuvenate Your Body in 40 Days

This is an old recipe and a potent mixture, based on only two ingredients. The first one is fig, an extremely good fruit for health, both fresh and dry. The best figs are those of a light, yellow colour. During the drying process, their healing properties multiply. The fig's natural proteins and sugars are easy to metabolise. Dried figs can significantly increase energy production, improve our mental activity, our mood and capacity to work.

Dried figs are also very rich in fibre, giving you a feeling of being full for a long time and improving digestion. They contain magnesium, iron, calcium and vitamin B. There is also a high amount of pectin in figs, which makes it an effective remedy for healing connective tissues, especially after joint and bone trauma. Another important component found in dried figs, rutin, works to strengthen capillaries.

> **"Dried figs can significantly increase energy production, improve our mental activity, our mood and capacity to work."**

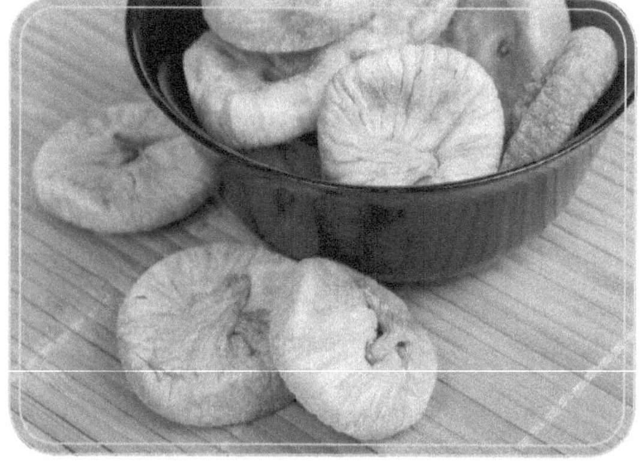

Daily consumption of figs decreases the risk of developing cardiovascular conditions. The following recipe is age-old and has been used in various cultures for the rejuvenation of the body, the improvement of its physical and mental abilities and as a treatment for many ailments. The recipe is extremely simple—take 20 dried figs, cut each of them in two and place them in a glass jar. Add olive oil, covering the figs, plus ½ - 1 cm above. Refrigerate for 40 days and then it will be ready to use. Simply eat half a fig and take a teaspoon of the oil from the jar 5-10 minutes before breakfast. Continue until finished. You will feel the healing power of the remedy straight away. Repeat this 2-3 times a year.

Great News on Coughing and Chocolate

Professor Alyn Morice from the University of Hull, a specialist of cardiovascular and respiratory diseases, and his team proved that the best remedy for coughing is chocolate—specifically darker varieties with a high content of cocoa and low sugar content. The results evidently confirmed that cocoa works better than any other cough mixtures. So, the scientists recommend eating dark chocolate regularly to help ease your cough symptoms.

The key substance responsible for this result is Theobromine, found in cocoa beans. It suppresses coughs even more effectively than Codeine, which is the main component in many cough mixtures. To maximise the effect, melt the chocolate so it becomes a warm liquid. The hot chocolate helps to create a protective membrane in your throat. However, even a piece of chocolate will bring relief if you keep it in your mouth until it has completely melted.

Garlic Husk—Look Younger for Longer

Don't throw your white garlic husk away—save it. It's one of the most valuable natural aids for longevity. If you drink a special concoction made of white garlic husk you will feel and look your best. So, what is it about garlic husk? What are its healing properties?

If you look at a small piece of husk under a microscope you can see Quercetin crystals neatly laid in rows. Studies show that the garlic husk contains 4 percent of the powerful antioxidant, bioflavonoid Quercetin. This is a natural, biologically active substance belonging to the vitamin R group. Quercetin is now a very popular supplement that can be found in garlic, onion, apple

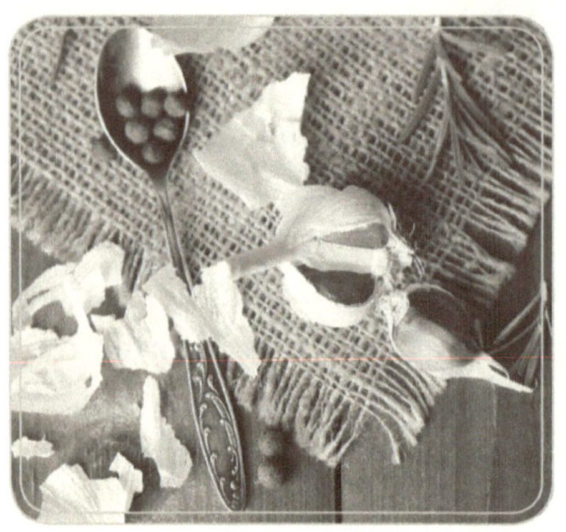

and green tea. It is available as a supplement in health shops and chemists. However, making your own solution costs almost nothing and you can be sure it's purely natural.

The famous Dr Atkins considered Quercetin to be the best antihistamine and prescribed it to his patients suffering from various allergies. However, Quercetin is even more popular as a preventive means for cardiovascular conditions. People who take a lot of Quercetin have a lower risk of heart attacks, strokes and blood clots forming. We can prepare two different drinks based on garlic that are beneficial in many ways.

Garlic Husk Drink

To prepare this drink, take 4 glasses of water, bring to the boil and allow cool for 3 minutes. Then take 4 handfuls of garlic husk and cover with the hot water. Leave for 6-8 hours. It is best to drink all 4 glasses in one day, or at least as much as you feel you can drink. Do this for 10 days in a row and the difference will be visible. Your skin will become smoother, radiant and younger looking. Remember, what we see externally is also happening inside the body.

Garlic And Lemon Water

This recipe is an ancient Chinese homoeopathic remedy and has been found recorded on five-thousand-year-old clay tablets. This amazing solution cleanses the body of excess fat, bad cholesterol and calcium deposits, dramatically improving metabolism. Blood vessels become non-rigid, which works to prevent heart attacks, angina, sclerosis and tumour formation. But that's not all—it can ease headaches and tinnitus and improve vision.

Peel one whole garlic bulb but don't remove the tiny, thin membranes from the cloves. Wash one lemon with boiling water and remove its rind. Put the prepared garlic and lemon rind into a blender and mix well. Put it in a glass container and cover with 600g of cooled, boiled water. Close the lid and refrigerate for 3-4 days. Then strain the tincture and take 50g of it on an empty stomach in the morning every day for 3 months. Then take a break for a month. If you follow this recipe exactly and take it regularly you will feel your body's rejuvenation.

A Killer of Extra Kilos

This is a mixture of common ingredients that burn excess fat.

- 4 cloves of garlic

- 4 small tomatoes

- 1 glass of water

- 6 ice cubes (optional)

- 6 tablespoons of lemon juice

Put all ingredients in a blender and mix well. Take this mixture 2-3 times a week, half an hour after breakfast. Lycopene in tomatoes is a strong antioxidant that helps in removing excess fat, toxins and other impurities from your body. The amazing properties of garlic are also great for burning calories and improving your general well-being. The mixture works its best when we observe our diet and try to avoid sugar.

The Plant of "Eternal Youth"

Plants have been used in folk medicine for centuries for their incredible healing properties. One, in particular, can decrease sugar levels, cleanse the kidneys, rejuvenate skin and stop hair loss, as well as treating respiratory conditions such as:

- Pneumonia
- Sore throat
- Asthma
- Seasonal allergies

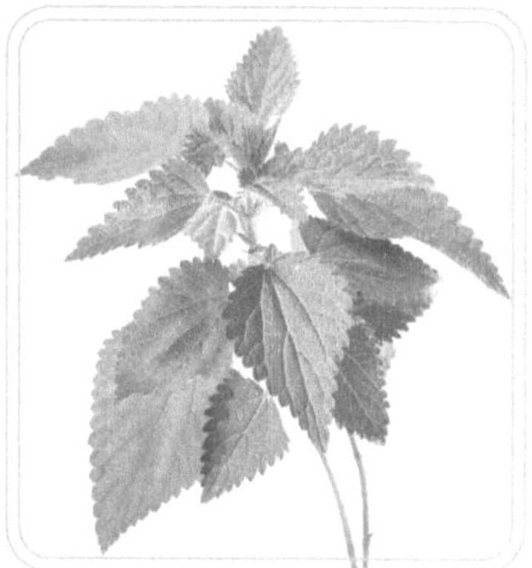

This plant, with its rich scope of healing applications, is *nettle*—let's see what it's useful for.

SKIN: Nettle tea has antibacterial, nutritional, cleansing and stimulating effects on the skin. It also supports collagen production. This tea can be drunk with honey or used externally for rinsing your face, as an ingredient for facial masks or for making nettle ice.

KIDNEYS: Nettle is a great diuretic and detoxifies the kidneys. It is also said that nettle tea can prevent the formation of kidney stones.

HAIR: It prevents hair loss, treats dandruff and makes hair stronger and brighter.

BLOOD CIRCULATION: As nettle is rich in chlorophyll, it helps to control bad cholesterol and improves blood circulation.

DIABETES: Nettle tea works to decrease the sugar in your blood.

PROSTATE: It works against hyperplasia, or enlargement of the prostate. Nettle cleanses the prostate and prevents cancer.

This list could be expanded to include immune system support, fighting anaemia and fatigue, insomnia and stress-related conditions. All the varieties of nettle available are medicinal.

To make nettle tea is simple. Bring 1 litre of pure water to the boil, add 1 tablespoon of dry nettle leaves and cover with a lid for at least 10 minutes. Then percolate, add honey if desired and drink up to 3 cups a day. You can also add some lemon and mint for better taste. Using nettle tea regularly is very beneficial in many ways.

Parsley Lotion

This home-made lotion with parsley eliminates acne, reduces any kind of swelling or irritation, whitens, tones and refreshes the skin. It can also remove freckles. This lotion could also be a great supplement in treating kidney disease and diabetes, as well as inflammation, by consuming a teaspoon before each meal.

Ingredients:

- 2 tablespoons of chopped parsley leaves.

- 1 teaspoon of lemon juice or apple cider vinegar.

- 200ml of water.

Preparation:

- Boil parsley in water for 15 minutes.

- Let it cool down and add the lemon juice or apple cider vinegar—your choice.

- Keep in a glass container in the fridge.

How to use it:

Simply apply it where needed using your fingers. Do it regularly, at least twice a day. It takes a bit of time to see the results, as is often the case with natural remedies.

Flax Seeds Against Parasites

Flax seeds could be considered the undiscovered champion of anti-parasite treatments. Flax seeds' decoction cleanses the body of almost all parasites—apart from Ascaris. However, if you add in a couple of cloves, even Ascaris won't survive. Flaxseed oil is also a popular product with a specific odour and a lot of health benefits.

Mix 2 tablespoons of flax seeds with one litre of water. Leave to simmer for 30 minutes, then leave to continue infusing until cooled down. Then take between 100 and 200ml half an hour before meals 2-3 times a day. Don't be tempted to sweeten the concoction for the period of cleansing. Sugar will only reduce its efficacy.

Whole flax seeds can be used to rid the body of parasites, by consuming 2 tablespoons of seeds twice a day for 8-10 days. They can be also used preventatively.

The Healing Power of Coriander

One of the best natural products to remove mercury and other heavy metals from your body is a herb known as coriander or cilantro. Fresh coriander contains large amounts of Vitamins A, B, C, E, K and PP, as well as potassium, calcium, manganese, iron, phosphorus, pectin, rutin, alkaloids and essential oils.

Because of such natural richness, coriander is known for its anti-inflammatory, anti-bacterial, life-force strengthening, detoxifying and soothing properties. Featuring it in your diet plays a preventative role against infectious and viral illnesses. Coriander also supports cardiovascular, nervous and respiratory systems, as well as the health of the digestive tract.

Get into the habit of adding fresh coriander to your meals. Coriander essential oil is also a very powerful anti-inflammatory and detoxifying substance. You only need 1-2 drops of it in a glass of water every day to have an effect. Research has confirmed that doing this for six weeks can help the body get rid of up to 80% of heavy metals and toxins.

Warning: as always, consult your doctor before using any of these natural remedies.

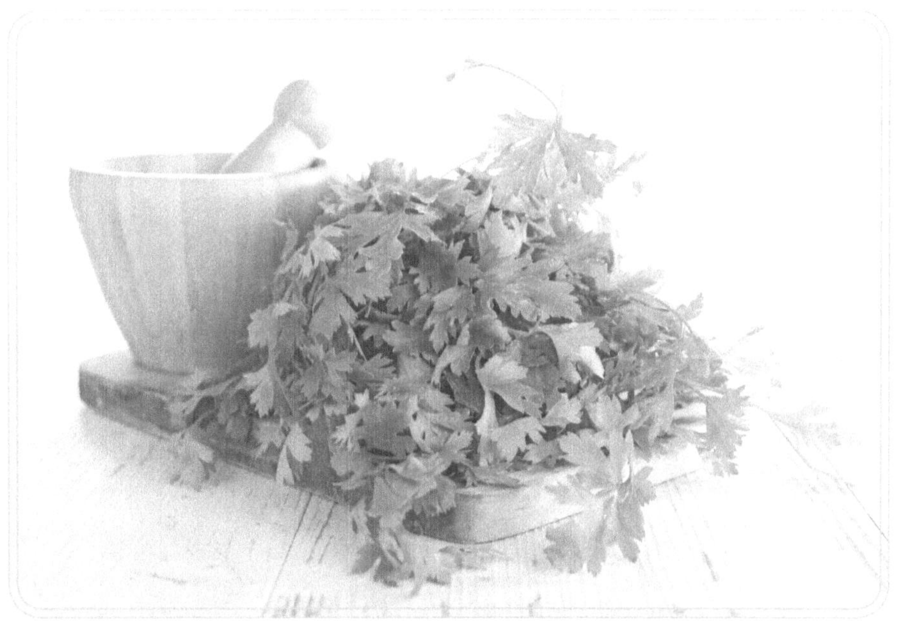

GOLDEN AGE—THE SECRET OF LONGEVITY

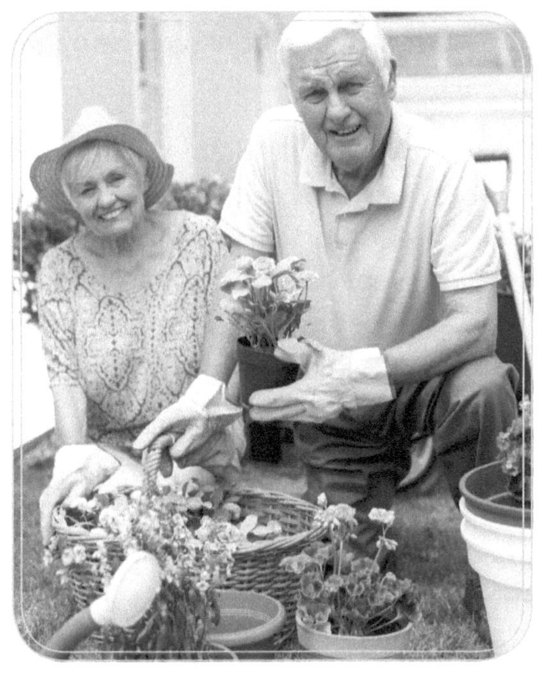

> "There is no magic bullet when it comes to ageing well but I can tell you from personal experience that the process of ageing need not be a bad thing."

There is no magic bullet when it comes to ageing well but I can tell you from personal experience that the process of ageing need not be a bad thing.

Living through our golden years, we don't have a lot of time to waste. However, we still have plenty of time to live and enjoy our life. We need to live our quality time with gusto, not spending it doing nothing.

Centenarians, as a rule, are happy and optimistic human beings. They have extremely low rates of depression and other psychiatric problems, suggesting that personality traits may be one of the most significant factors in longevity. However, happiness doesn't mean you can completely disregard the basics: nutrition, water, exercise and sleep.

The better you treat your body throughout your life, the better your ageing experience will be. A team of researchers at UCLA showed that people with a deep sense of happiness and well-being had lower levels of inflammatory conditions and stronger antiviral and antibody responses.

Researchers at UNSW's Centre for Healthy Brain Ageing did examine 345 people aged between 95 and 106. Co-director Perminder Sachdev said, "One important finding was that these individuals have often been very healthy until a very late age. If they have diseases such as hypertension, coronary artery disease, diabetes, often these are late in developing."

"Those who avoided disease were probably genetically blessed," Professor Sachdev continued, "while those with delayed onset of disease have had good lifestyles." Then he added, "The seeds for healthy old age are sown very early in life, with a good education. Achieving healthy old age is actually a lifelong enterprise. You're really looking at your risk factors, your diet, your weight, your exercise, cognitive activity."

Donna Bauer, organiser of the Century Club celebrations for centenarians, at their recent gathering at Government House in Melbourne pointed out, "Reaching 100 is such an incredible milestone, so worth celebrating," she said. "For other centenarians to meet people born in the same year is just so valuable for them. They're full of positivity, great advice and always love sharing their secrets to longevity."

Dan Buettner, the author of *Blue Zones*, took a map and highlighted five small geographical areas in the world where the population outlives the Americans and Western Europeans by around a decade on average. They are Okinawa in Japan, Ikaria island in Greece, Sardinia in Italy, the Nicoya in Costa Rica and Loma Linda in California.

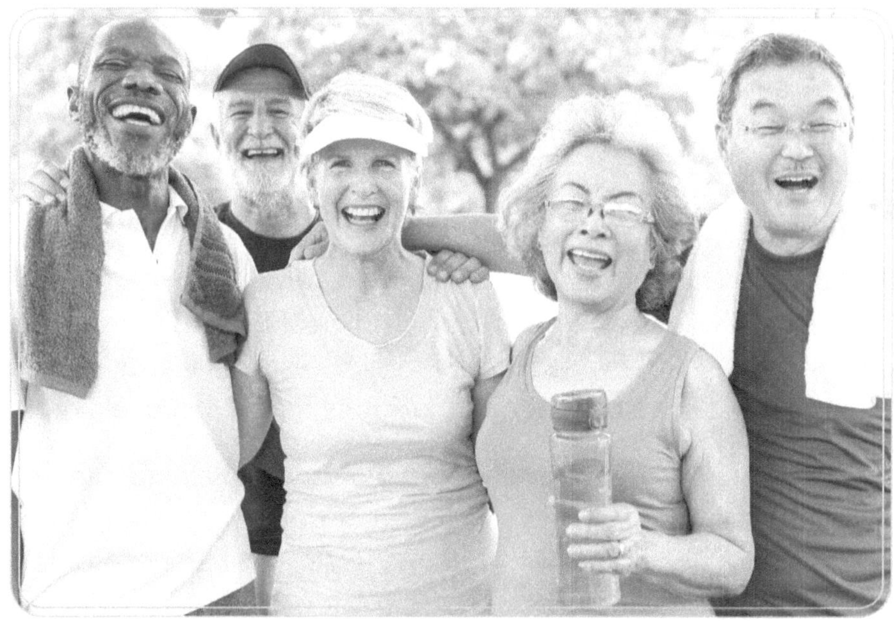

Everybody has heard about Okinawans exceptional longevity with the largest number of centenarians per capita on the planet. There have been a tremendous number of studies into the Okinawa diet, its water, etc. But are those the only explanations for its citizens' long lives? Older Okinawans readily articulate the reason they get up in the morning. They call it "ikigai", which means "a reason for being". That implies clear roles of responsibility and feelings of being needed.

At 103, Ushi Okushima has just got her first job, selling oranges at the market. "She has farmed her whole life, but she has never had a job where she got a salary," says Canadian scientist Craig

Willcox. "She is so excited about her first job. It is her 'ikigai' at the moment".

Let now move to Ikaria, in Greece, otherwise known as "the island of long life". Evangelia Karnava, who has lived in Ikaria all her life, was born in 1916. She radiates a fierce energy and she is an important person for her three children, seven grandchildren, four great-grandchildren and her great-great-grandchild. "I'm going to live to be 115, they need me," she says. "My grand-mother was 107."

Our next stop brings us to Sardinia, Italy. Zelinda Paglieno, who turned 102 in October, offers not-so-sobering advice when asked for the secret to her long and healthy life: "I've never smoked, but a little wine is good for you—and that's something I still do now. We have very good grapes here," she explained.

"I'm not old!" Caterina Moi exclaims after explaining she was born in 1920. She still hears well, can negotiate the steep steps to her first-floor home with relative ease and has no problem recounting past moments in her life. Her advice: "Two fingers width of red wine—and no more—at lunchtime every day."

In Nicoya, Costa Rica, centenarians believe in "Plan de Vida" which translates to "plan for life". Successful centenarians there have a strong sense of purpose. They feel needed and want to contribute to society. Old Miguel Costa, 104 years old, admits: "When I wake up in the morning I have a plan for the day. And for the week and for the next year. I do useful things for my family and neighbours and that keeps me going".

Now to the US, whose longest-living people reside in Loma Linda, California. Out of 22,000 residents, as many as a third of them are Seventh-day Adventists. Their faith instructs them to treat their bodies as temples: no smoking or alcohol, little or no meat or fish, plenty of exercise and—most importantly—a sense of purpose.

At 100 years old, Benita Welebir says: "I am extremely energetic, but I also believe in full rest. If you have full rest, you can go like a little speedster." What's extraordinary about her longevity is that it's not out of the ordinary. In Loma Linda, Benita is just another active older person. One of her neighbours at the Linda Valley Villa is 101, another is 100 and several belong to the 95-plus club. Welebir continues: "I've always been happy and if I'm sad, I know I'll be happy again."

Apart from those five Blue Zones, we see centenarians in many other countries and places. They are also happy to voice their opinions on longevity. People in Siberia and the Chechen Republic are well-known for their endurance and resilience and some of them live long lives. Here's just a handful of their wise words:

- "My secret to a longer life? I never get angry at anyone!"

- "Reading good books prolongs life."

- "Find what you love to do. Then, even turning 100, I can say my life begins afresh."

- "Get out of your car and walk instead."

- "To live long, one must work hard all their life."

- "My secret—every day I drink 30g of vodka mixed with sunflower oil."

- "Every day, eat a carrot, without fail."

Now we go back to the States where Lucille Lewis, 100 years old and from Kentucky, formulates her viewpoint: "Life is a joy. You are not obliged to feel happy all the time, but you have to be satisfied with your life." Another 100-year-old woman from New York, Ruth, added: "Dress elegantly every day of your life."

There are more people than ever aged 100 years of age and older in Australia and a new study has found that as a group they need less home care than far younger seniors. If anyone embodies that spirit, it is 100-year-old Bert Bush, who lives on Victoria's Mornington Peninsula. "I want to live life now that I'm 100 years of age," he said. "I know I can't live like a 20-year-old, but I still want to live life."

If there is a secret to a long life, centenarian Denise Johnston agrees it's not complicated: "I sort of don't worry about things too much," she said.

An Australian centenarian of Hungarian descent Antal Torok, born in January 1914, when asked what helped him reach such an impressive age, stated that his loving family and keeping mentally and physically active were the key. He only recently gave up driving, but continued reading, cooking and cleaning. He said he is very much interested in local as well as world affairs. "You have to be not overdoing things, but always doing something," he said.

Well. By now, you, my reader, have already learnt these secrets. The ones that I presented to you as the fundamental systems for longevity. Those, in a way, have been confirmed by real centenarians' opinions from across the globe.

The only thing left to do is implementing the systems, strategies and tactics recommended, if you like them. Please let me know how you get on and let's celebrate our achievements together. I wish you all the best from the bottom of my heart.

You can always contact me via my website
www.lukinlongevity.com, and also by Messenger, Skype,
WhatsApp or Viber, and other social media.

LIGHTS, CAMERA ACTION!

Lights: your System of Beliefs,
enlightened and illuminated…

Camera: your System of Goals with
focus, precision and exposure…

Action: your System of Actions:
Do it now—don't procrastinate…

Your film is rolling.

www.ingramcontent.com/pod-product-compliance
Lightning Source LLC
Chambersburg PA
CBHW051309250726
48656CB00004B/1554